BREAKING OUT

A Woman's Guide
to Coping With Acne
at Any Age

—◀◉▶—

LYDIA PRESTON

A FIRESIDE BOOK
PUBLISHED BY SIMON & SCHUSTER
New York   London   Toronto   Sydney

This publication contains the opinions and ideas of its author. It is intended to provide helpful and informative material on the subjects addressed in the publication.
It is sold with the understanding that the author and publisher are not engaged in
rendering medical, health, or any other kind of personal professional services in the
book. The reader should consult his or her medical, health, or other competent professional before adopting any of the suggestions in this book or drawing inferences
from it.

The author and publisher specifically disclaim all responsibility for any liability, loss,
or risk, personal or otherwise, which is incurred as a consequence, directly or indirectly, of the use and application of any of the contents of this book.

FIRESIDE
Rockefeller Center
1230 Avenue of the Americas
New York, NY 10020

FIRESIDE and colophon are registered trademarks
of Simon & Schuster, Inc.

For information about special discounts for bulk purchases,
please contact Simon & Schuster Special Sales at
1-800-456-6798 or business@simonandschuster.com.

Designed by Jan Pisciotta

Manufactured in the United States of America
1 3 5 7 9 10 8 6 4 2

Library of Congress Cataloging-in-Publication Data
Preston, Lydia.
Breaking out : a woman's guide to coping with acne at any age / Lydia Preston.
p.   cm.
Includes bibliographical references and index.
1. Acne—Popular works. 2. Women—Diseases—Popular works. I. Title.
RL131.P746 2004
616.5'3—dc22   2004045221
ISBN 0-7432-3623-8

For
Gloria Norris
&
Jimmy, Will, and Blair Hicks
With love and gratitude for their patience and support

ACKNOWLEDGMENTS

This book could never have been written without the generous help of the many dermatologists who patiently listened to my countless questions and answered them with such forbearance and clarity:

Tina Alster, M.D.; Wilma Bergfeld, M.D.; Susan Bershad, M.D.; Diane Berson, M.D.; Fredric Brandt, M.D.; Harold Brody, M.D.; Cheryl Burgess, M.D.; Anthony Chu, M.D.; Mark Dahl, M.D.; William Danby, M.D.; Alan Dattner, M.D.; Richard Fried, M.D., Ph.D.; Karen Grossman, M.D.; Richard Glogau, M.D.; Debra Jaliman, M.D.; Albert M. Kligman, M.D., Ph.D.; Elizabeth McBurney, M.D.; Marianne O'Donoghue, M.D.; Norman Orentreich, M.D.; David Orentreich, M.D.; Lawrence Parrish, M.D.; Gary Peck, M.D.; Nicholas Perricone, M.D.; Gerd Plewig, M.D.; Laurie Polis, M.D.; Howard Pride, M.D.; Vail Reese, M.D.; Katie Rodan, M.D.; Deborah Sarnoff, M.D.; Alan Shalita, M.D.; Robert Silverman, M.D.; Susan Taylor, M.D.; Robert Weiss, M.D.; Patricia Wexler, M.D.; Julie Winfield, M.D.; John Yarborough, M.D.

Many thanks also to:

Diane Ackley, Paula Begoun, Bobbi Brown, Greg Estrada, Sandy Gordon, John Kuleza, Ken Klein, Eileen Leach, Ken Marenous, Erin Nieman, Anthony Simion, Shirley Weinstein.

And at the American Academy of Dermatology: Donna Stein, Karen Sideris, and Missy Lundberg.

Contents

Acknowledgments

Introduction *by Tina Alster, M.D.*   XI

Chapter One
Facing Up to Acne   1

Chapter Two
Breaking Free   11

Chapter Three
Understanding Acne   18

Chapter Four
"Will It Make Me Break Out?"   34

Chapter Five
Over-the-Counter Remedies   46

Chapter Six
Prescription Treatment   66

Chapter Seven
Accutane   90

Chapter Eight
Hormones and Hormonal Treatment   106

Chapter Nine

Herbs, Homeopathy, and Other Alternatives   121

Chapter Ten

The Mind-Skin Connection   139

Chapter Eleven

Looking Good   147

Chapter Twelve

Acne and Your Children   163

Chapter Thirteen

Scars and Scar Revision   175

Chapter Fourteen

Healing the Inner Scars   196

Appendix A

Acne Drugs in Pregnancy   201

Appendix B

Resources   205

Bibliography   215

Index   227

Introduction

————⟨◇⟩————

by Tina Alster, M.D.

Acne is an elusive and resourceful foe. It is stubborn, with a remarkable ability to shrug off the most aggressive medical treatments. It is unpredictable, adept at appearing or disappearing without rhyme or reason. And it is malicious, capable of inflicting terrible damage in the form of physical scars that disfigure the face and emotional wounds that lacerate the psyche.

Most of the women who come to my office with acne or acne scarring have spent years battling this tenacious adversary. They are fed up with embarrassing breakouts and with remedies that haven't worked for them. Many are devastated by the facial scarring that confronts them each time they look into a mirror or catch sight of their reflection in a store window. And they all are sick and tired of waiting for it to just go away. Even though adult acne is a common phenomenon, with as many as half of all women experiencing at least occasional flare-ups, most of my female acne patients can scarcely believe that they are still breaking out in their twenties and thirties, let alone their forties and fifties!

A few years ago, writer Lydia Preston was one of these patients—frustrated by years of fighting acne, and desperately unhappy about the scars on her face. These were experiences that she soon drew on when, after undergoing several surgical procedures to repair the scars, she collaborated with me on a book about my specialty, cosmetic laser surgery. I can safely say I have never met a journalist or researcher who became more thoroughly immersed in any subject.

Lydia spent hours watching me and the other dermatologists in my office at work—and then spent many more hours grilling each of us about what she had observed. She interviewed my nurses and aestheticians—and even my office manager. She pored over medical journals and textbooks. She attended dermatology meetings to hear other specialists lecture. And she sat down for long, heart-to-heart conversations with dozens of my patients—many of them other acne sufferers—gaining the kind of insight into their emotional and practical concerns that busy physicians rarely have the time to explore.

It is clear that she has brought the same dedication and passion for detail to this book about acne in women. As any dermatologist will instantly recognize from the names cited in the text, she has interviewed many of the world's leading acne experts—true giants of dermatology, whose research constitutes the foundation for modern acne treatment. She has similarly sought out renowned authorities on acne scarring and scar treatment, on cosmetics and cosmetic chemistry, on alternative therapies, and on the psychological ramifications of skin disease.

The result is a uniquely comprehensive examination of the myriad complexities of acne and the confusing welter of treatment options. The book's exceptionally clear explanations of how acne occurs and how different remedies work or don't work to eliminate acne should come as a revelation to anyone frustrated by years of persistent treatment failure. It will certainly be a source of reassurance and wisdom to which any woman can turn with confidence at any time when an acne outbreak occurs—whether she is exasperated by periodic flares or heartsick over disfiguring cysts or scars.

How do you sort through the hundreds of competing over-the-counter acne preparations that now crowd drugstore, supermarket, and department store shelves to zero in on the handful that are likely to be most effective for you? How do you avoid things that make acne worse? How can you work with a dermatologist to get the most out of prescription acne medicines? Treatments frequently fail simply because patients are not fully informed about how to use them correctly. What can you do to ensure that your medicines will work as they are supposed to? How will you cope with any side effects that may occur? And what steps do you take if your condition changes, as acne-prone skin inevitably does with age, or the hormonal shifts of pregnancy, menstruation, menopause, or any of a dozen other reasons?

What about acne scarring? Even very mild or occasional breakouts have the potential to leave permanent scars, and despite numerous exciting innovations in dermatologic surgery, these mutilating rents in the fabric of the skin remain among the most daunting challenges that face any cosmetic surgeon. In many instances, the most effective techniques are also the riskiest ones. How do you weigh the relative risks and benefits? How do you find a qualified practitioner who will employ the best and safest methods for your skin type—and for the types of scars you have?

Finally, how do you heal the inner scars of acne? Countless studies testify to its damaging emotional impact. How does any woman get past those feelings to get over acne once and for all and move on with her life?

Breaking Out addresses those questions, and many more, with information drawn from Lydia's own experience with acne and the toll it takes, her years of reporting on dermatology, and her sympathetic exploration into other patients' concerns. I know it will be invaluable to all of my acne patients, and I look forward to recommending it to them.

Dr. Tina Alster, clinical professor of dermatology at Georgetown University, is director of the Washington Institute of Dermatologic Laser Surgery and consulting dermatologist for Lancôme, luxury products division of L'Oréal USA, Inc.

Chapter One

———◦———

Facing Up to Acne

THIS IS THE BOOK I've always wished I had for myself.

I have had acne, off and on, most of my life. From the time I was fourteen until I was in my mid-thirties, there wasn't a single day when I had perfectly clear skin. Sometimes it was very badly broken out; at other times it was marked by just a pimple or two. But for more than twenty years, it was never totally clear.

In more recent years, the breakouts have come and gone. There have been months when I haven't had a single blemish, only to have one or two, or a small crop, pop up seemingly out of nowhere. Infuriatingly, they have never failed to appear at major life events—job interviews, my wedding, the birth of my children.

In all those years, I could never find a book, magazine article, or doctor's pamphlet that answered all of the questions I had or that gave me all of the information I needed to clear up my skin and keep it clear. When I turned to dermatologists for answers, few had the time, in the course of a typical perfunctory office visit, to even fill in the blanks.

It wasn't until I began writing about skin as a journalist and started reading about acne in medical textbooks, listening to lectures at dermatology conventions, and interviewing medical experts, that I at last began to truly understand why my skin kept breaking out, why it made me feel so terrible, and what I could do about it.

This book is the result. It is written for women like me— young women plagued by breakouts into their twenties, thirties, and beyond; working women, wives, and mothers who thought they were safely past the age of acne yet now are astonished and dismayed to find their faces breaking out like teenagers'; and older women still battling those maddening eruptions even as they face the challenges and changes that come with advancing age—yes, including menopause.

THE NEW "WOMAN'S DISEASE"

No grown woman expects to have acne. At any age. I certainly never did. The conviction that acne is purely a teenage disease—something that you quickly outgrow—is among the most widely held of the many misconceptions that surround this most common of skin conditions.

"Women come in here held captive to that myth all the time," says New York dermatologist Laurie Polis, who estimates that as many as 70 percent of her women patients complain to some degree about breakouts. "And they all say, 'Why am I getting *this*? I'm too old. I'm thirty-four!' "

"For the most part they are shocked that they still have it," agrees Dr. Marianne O'Donoghue, associate professor of dermatology at Rush-Presbyterian–St. Luke's Medical Center in Chicago. O'Donoghue says that fully half of her acne patients are women between the ages of twenty and fifty. "And they all somehow think that on the eve of their twenty-first birthday, their acne should have magically disappeared."

But that is far from the case.

These days, dermatologists are as likely to characterize acne as a woman's disease as a teenager's. In fact, the number of women seeking medical care for acne has increased so dramatically in recent years that some doctors actually refer to the phenomenon as an "epidemic."

"I've been a dermatologist for fifty-five years, and when I began, we were all taught that acne was an adolescent disease," says Dr. Albert M. Kligman, professor emeritus of dermatology at the University of Pennsylvania and the one of the preeminent acne researchers of the twentieth century. "We all said, 'Just wait; it will go away.' Well, that is no longer the case."

A LINGERING PREDICAMENT

Acne is of course, the all-but-inevitable rite of adolescent passage. Almost everyone gets some form of it, even if it's just an occasional small pimple or two, between the ages of twelve and twenty. In general, teenage boys usually suffer from the worst forms, probably because males produce more androgens, the hormones that play a key role in stimulating breakouts. Acne in teenage girls tends to be more of a slow-burning, smoldering disease. However, it is much more likely to be long lasting. Most boys eventually outgrow their acne; many girls never do.

"At least 30 percent of women who have significant acne—that is, pimple acne, not just blackheads—in their twenties, will continue to have acne into their thirties, forties, and fifties," says Kligman. In fact, studies have shown that for women who still have, or who acquire, acne in their twenties, the mean duration is twenty years. Some will still be breaking out in their seventies and eighties.

Adult acne is actually not a new phenomenon. "There are persons who suffer from acne all their days," observed nineteenth-century Viennese physician Ferdinand Hebra, the leading European dermatologist of his era. And even today, doctors disagree over whether the incidence of acne among women is actually on the rise, or if the numbers merely reflect the fact that appearance-conscious Western women are more likely than their grandmothers to seek treatment from dermatologists.

Hard statistics are difficult to come by, but according to two surveys conducted at England's University of Leeds, a major center of acne research, the incidence of serious acne in women rose from 10 percent in 1979 to 14 percent in 1996. Mild acne jumped from 35 percent to 54 percent over the same seventeen-year period, suggesting that more than half of women today suffer from at least occasional or periodic break-outs. In 1998, Neutrogena, one of the leading U.S. makers of nonprescription acne products, conducted its own survey and learned that 59 percent of women between the ages of twenty-five and thirty-nine had suffered from acne in the previous year. According to one market research firm, more prescription and over-the-counter acne medications are now sold to adults than to teens.

If acne is indeed on the rise among women, there is no conclusive evidence to tell us why. The most frequently fingered suspect is stress, although there have been no smoking-gun research findings that definitively connect stress and acne.

"There are no good studies," concedes Kligman. "But I see it all the time in the histories I take. It's professional women—doctors, lawyers, and executives—who come in with acne. This may be lousy science, but it's good empirical medicine."

But haven't women always had to cope with stress? What about, say, colonial women, battling the frontier, scratching crops out of rocky fields, bearing children and losing them to infant diseases?

"In colonial times you didn't have your e-mail, your telephone, your Palm Pilot, and everybody constantly trying to get a hold of you," says San Francisco dermatologist Katie Rodan, cocreator of the top-selling Proactiv acne products. "You can't escape the tensions of modern-day life. Sure, part of the demand for treatment is that more women are out in the workplace and are more concerned about their looks, so they're seeking help. But I think the stresses of modern life are responsible for a lot of dermatological problems, and acne is no exception."

Kligman agrees. "My grandparents came from Russia. And life was hard for those women. They bore a lot of children. They were poor and went to bed tired every night from working all day. But I don't think they were under the kinds of stresses that produce acne. They had hardships, but they didn't have the same emotional stress. My guess is that arduous living, which is the case for 90 percent of the world's population, doesn't produce acne. But, you get into the American situation, where you're running all damn day long, and you're a soccer mom and you have a job, and are trying to juggle all that stuff. Well, then, God help you, because I don't know who the hell else will."

GETTING HELP

Happily, there has never been a better time to find help—whether it is for the lone pimple that pops up each month like clockwork just before your menstrual period, or the raging conflagrations of inflamed lesions that can disfigure the face with physical scars and lacerate the psyche with painful emotional wounds. Today, there are numerous over-the-counter treatments that can stop mild or transient acne in its tracks, as well as potent prescription medicines that can successfully combat severe or recalcitrant acne. There is even a burgeoning new segment of the skin-care industry devoted to the persistent flare-ups of adult women.

Most of these remedies were undreamed of when my own acne was at its worst. I saw a succession of dermatologists over the years, and when their pastes and lotions, their dry ice treatments, their light therapies and their antibiotics (not to mention all the cleansers, ointments, steam treatments, vitamin supplements, face masks, and other stuff I tried on my own) failed to work, all they had to offer was the thin reassurance that the only real cure for my acne was "Tincture of Time." In other words, it would eventually go away on its own.

Only it didn't. In the end, it wasn't the passage of time that finally cured my acne. It was Accutane—the strong prescription medicine that first became available in the 1980s. And even then, I can't say I was truly "cured." I have acne-prone skin, which essentially means that my skin is poised to break out at the drop of hat—although never again to the painfully obvious or destructive degree it did before.

Accutane represents the crowning achievement of a kind of golden age in acne research and drug development that began in the 1960s, after centuries in which remedies were based largely on folklore and guesswork.

These days, armed with an abundance of proven treatments based on a foundation of continuing research, no dermatologist—or knowledgeable medical professional of any specialty—has to counsel an acne patient to just wait it out. Experts say that now no one should have to live with acne or its consequences for very long.

"It's clear we have made enormous progress, and I assert that today, almost 100 percent of patients with acne can be well managed, if not cured," says Kligman. "This proves what we said forty years ago, that it's time to learn something about this disease, and now as a result of forty years of research—not talk, not speculation—we are finally competent to diagnose it and treat it."

So why do you still have acne? Which you presumably do if you picked up this book and have read this far. Why does anyone? How can that be, if there are so many good ways to get rid of it?

WHY ACNE TREATMENTS FAIL

The very abundance of remedies is part of the problem. Not only are the many choices confusing (How do you pick?), but it is axiomatic in medicine that if there are many different treatments for any given condition, there isn't one that can be counted on to be surefire. That is very much the case with acne. It is not a simple disease, and it does not yield to simple solutions.

Acne is what doctors call a "multifactorial" and "pleomorphic" disease. That means that it has multiple causes and manifests itself in many different ways. Successful long-term treatment generally demands that several, if not all, of the causes be addressed simultaneously. Most cases are best treated with a combination of several medications, and it can take a lot of trial and error to devise a successful strategy to fit any one person's individual set of circumstances.

For any doctor, coming up with the right solution for any specific patient can entail a surprising amount of medical spadework, as Polis says she learned as a young dermatology resident.

"When I was a resident, everybody got assigned something called a basic science project," she recalls. "My basic science project was acne. And I thought, 'Ah-ha! This is going to be easy!' I mean, *acne*? How hard could that be? Well! I had to research and research and *research*. There are dozens of acne medicines out there, and you can't just pick a few out of the hat. You have to match each one to the type of acne. You have to match it to the severity of acne. You have to match it to the patient's lifestyle. Is she actually going to *use* whatever you give her? A lot of patients don't, because it irritates them. Or they think it's not working. Or both. So you have to know every feature of every drug you use. Does it work in the daytime? Does it leave a residue? Is it going to dry her out? Or turn her red? Can she wear it under makeup? It's just incredibly hard to get it all right."

Acne experts emphasize that successful acne treatment is as much an art as a science, and just as there is no single recipe for success, none can be relied on to be successful in every case. Dismayingly, grown women are particularly hard to treat. In a 1998 study of adult women with persistent acne, 88 percent of the study subjects saw no improvement at all when given oral antibiotics, one of the standard workhorses of acne treatment. And a full 33 percent did not respond to the powerful acne drug Accutane, widely regarded as a virtual cure for most of the patients who take it.

"Post-adolescent acne in women is tough," warns Kligman. "It's not like the pimples that kids get, that heal up in a week. Women get these crops of lesions in the lower part of the face. They are deeper and more diffuse than teenagers'. They keep coming back, they stay there for weeks at a time, they leave scars. And they are very, very difficult to treat."

He adds: "I suspect the majority of dermatologists don't have the time—or the inclination—to take care of these patients. They take out their prescription pads and say, 'Here's your tetracycline. Here's your Retin-A. Good-bye.' Well, that may work for some of these young kids with acne, but for the kind of acne that most women have—the persistent cases—it's never going to work."

YOU HAVE THE POWER

According to dermatologists, one of the keys to effective acne therapy is knowledge—on the part of acne patients. "I find that a lot of women who come in here with acne have gotten poor results with treatments because they don't really understand them," comments New York dermatologic surgeon Deborah Sarnoff. "And in general, the less a patient understands about an acne medicine, the more disappointed she's going to be with it."

Unfortunately, misunderstanding and misinformation are rampant when it comes to acne. Very often patients don't employ medicines in the most effective ways because they haven't a clue as to how they are to be used. In many cases, that's because their doctors have been spectacularly unsuccessful in conveying important information about how different medicines work, how long they take, and how much persistence is required.

Moreover, the average brief office visit doesn't allow most doctors enough time to either thoughtfully devise or thoroughly explain any acne regimen—much less ones containing problematic medicines such as Retin-A, an acne treatment mainstay notorious for being both misunderstood and misused.

"Treating acne requires a lot of handholding," says San Francisco dermatologist Vail Reese. "Frankly, a lot of dermatologists try to avoid it because it can just be so frustrating."

And that is where I hope this book comes in. It is definitely not intended as a substitute for a dermatologist. I'm not a doctor, and I can't tell you which acne medicines are right for you, any more than I could write a prescription for one of them. Nor can I tell you exactly which choices to make when you're on your own, searching the increasingly crowded acne-treatment shelves at your drugstore or supermarket. But I hope I can give you information that will help you understand and use to best advantage any treatment you may employ—whether from a doctor or the drugstore. Your acne is not the same as your teenage son's, or your neighbor's, or even your own acne from ten years ago. Or ten days ago. And it probably cannot be treated in precisely the same way. The truth about acne is that there is no one acne prescription, no one acne cure for everyone.

"I always teach women, you have to be your own skin doctor/beauty expert, because no one can tell you exactly what to do or use all of the time—not even a skin doctor or a beauty expert," says celebrity makeup artist and cosmetics entrepreneur Bobbi Brown. "Your skin changes by the day, the season, the climate, your hormones. So you need to look and learn, and recognize when you need to be gentle, and when you need to be a little more aggressive. Or when you need to change something. I like to say you have to empower a person with a lot of knowledge and then she can make the decisions that are right for her."

And when it comes to acne, knowledge is definitely power.

Chapter Two

---◇---

Breaking Free

JUST AS KNOWLEDGE about acne treatments can empower you to banish breakouts, an understanding of its emotional effects can enable you to break its grip on your feelings.

Acne carries with it an inordinate weight of folkloric baggage that encumbers us to this day with wounding attitudes and perceptions. For centuries, no one had any idea what caused acne, and in the absence of hard information, a rich mythology rooted in conjecture and coincidence evolved to explain it.

Because acne typically makes its debut in adolescence—the time of sexual maturation—it seemed only natural to physicians of bygone days that it must somehow be connected with sex, or sexual misbehavior. Little children, innocent and presumably pure of thought, are also pure of skin. But with dawning sexuality and loss of innocence comes acne. It therefore followed that acne was somehow linked to sex, to sexual thoughts or masturbation or lewd behavior of some kind.

The oily appearance of acne-prone skin inspired another set of deductions. Lacking any real knowledge about the workings of the skin's oil-producing sebaceous glands, doctors long ago made the seemingly reasonable assumption that rich or greasy foods rendered the skin excessively oily and thus more prone to acne. Extending that logic, it only made sense that the more richly delicious the food, the more likely it would be to cause breakouts. That's the thinking that helped make chocolate a prime acne suspect—that and the coincidental fact that many women crave mood-elevating chocolate when they are under stress or before their menstrual periods, both of which can cause acne to flare.

An even more deeply ingrained myth is the belief that acne is caused by poor hygiene. Human beings seem to have a strong atavistic notion that skin disease is a mark of uncleanliness, some primitive sense that flawed skin is dirty skin. In acne, the appearance of blackheads—which can look very much like flecks of grime—only reinforces the conviction that external agents such as dirt or too much makeup bring on breakouts.

Dermatologists now know that none of these remarkably tenacious beliefs about sex, diet, and sanitation are true. Yet a whiff of immorality, a presumption of self-indulgence, and a suspicion of uncleanliness still cling to the condition of acne. Surveys show that fully three quarters of the general public believe that acne is caused either by poor hygiene or an unhealthy diet. Other than obesity, no other common medical condition carries such a burden of negative assumptions.

The result is that many women actually feel to blame for their own acne—an impression that may have been chiseled into their consciousness in early adolescence by parental admonitions to wash obsessively and steer clear of French fries.

"I find the most common assumption about acne is that it is a lifestyle disease," says acne specialist Dr. Susan Bershad, assistant clinical professor of dermatology at New York's Mount Sinai School of Medicine. "Women don't conceive of acne as a medical condition, but rather as something entirely under their control, like coloring their hair or getting in shape. If you read any teen magazine or women's magazine, you're constantly getting advice on how to treat acne as if it were something you can personally gain control over. But it's a medical condition, and it requires medical treatment."

Washington D.C. laser surgeon Dr. Tina Alster, who has treated hundreds of women for disfiguring acne scars, adds that one of the most striking common threads among these patients is the terrible sense of guilt that many of them feel. "They all feel they're being punished for something," says Alster. "On some level, every woman who has ever had acne thinks it's something she did. Or something she didn't do to herself."

THE "LAST HANDICAP"

As if hoary acne myths, misinformed magazine stories, and the painful memory of nagging parents weren't enough, apparently there are even deeper influences at work on the emotions of any person with acne, says Dr. Mark V. Dahl, chairman of the dermatology department at the University of New Mexico Medical School and founder of Camp Discovery, a summer camp for children with disfiguring skin conditions, most much more serious than acne. Says Dahl, "People with visible skin disease all feel a deep sense of shame."

Dahl calls skin disease "the last handicap"—a throwback to an earlier era in which victims of disease and disfigurement were routinely shunned or warehoused in institutions. Today, when AIDS patients rally by the thousands to demand research funding, when ordinary women go on television and candidly discuss their breast or cervical cancer, when TV host Katie Couric can take millions of Today show viewers on an endoscopic tour of her colon to highlight the importance of screening for rectal cancer, it would seem that no medical condition could too embarrassing, too difficult to discuss, or so dreadful that it must be hidden from view.

Skin disease is the all-too-common exception. People with severe eczema and psoriasis—or acne—don't rally or speak out. They hide. Or try to.

In interviews, women who have persistent acne say they feel a constant sense of embarrassment and shame. They see themselves as unattractive and believe that the first thing anyone notices about them is their bad skin. Yet they also sense that no one is very sympathetic to their plight.

Research confirms that double view. In a 1996 survey of attitudes toward acne, 98 percent of the respondents agreed that acne creates a negative impression. Yet, in a peculiar twist of logic, when asked, "Does acne have a negative effect on quality of life?" the same group overwhelmingly answered, "No."

Other studies show that because many people still erroneously believe acne is caused by poor hygiene or a bad diet, they regard acne sufferers as unclean or lacking in self-control. Studies dating back to the 1940s tell us that acne can be as stigmatizing as obesity. Like those who are overweight, people with chronic acne actually make less money over the course of a lifetime than those with clear skin. And just as overweight women are often perceived as deficient in willpower, women with acne may be viewed as careless about their personal hygiene or overindulgent in terms of their diet.

"You know, bad acne can be just as disfiguring as a birthmark," observed Emily, a forty-five-year-old real estate broker who had what she describes as real "pizza-face" acne into her late thirties. "But nobody looks at someone with a birthmark and thinks, 'Well, she doesn't wash her face enough.' I always wonder what kind of conclusions people are making about me based on my skin. I feel that they are judging me. That they look at me and think I'm some kind of slob."

NOBODY TALKS ABOUT IT

Given the fact that so many women find acne so embarrassing, if not deeply painful, it is probably small wonder that so few of them ever discuss it openly. Even so, I was surprised when I began interviewing other women with acne, and learned that everyone I spoke to had never talked about it at length to anyone, including doctors. In fact, most said they never talked about acne, period.

"I was in psychotherapy for more than twenty years, with three different therapists, and I never even talked about it to *my therapists*!" exclaimed Emily. "You know, you'd think the fact that I hated my own face would be pretty significant to a psychiatrist. But I went to three of them, and not one of them even brought it up." Of course, come to think of it, *I* never talked to anyone about *my* acne either. According to New York dermatologist Patricia Wexler, nobody does.

"No one 'embraces' their acne," says Wexler, who herself suffered from serious acne in her twenties. "A lot of people find it therapeutic to speak up about embarrassing personal problems or serious medical conditions. But nobody feels that way about acne."

I have a friend who doesn't have acne now, but the scars on her face bear eloquent witness to a ravaging bout in the past. She has said only one thing to me about it in all the years I have known her: "I won't talk about it. Ever."

IT'S NO JOKE

Sometimes it seems as if the only people who willingly bring up the subject of acne are comedians. On Valentine's Day, late-night host Jay Leno gleefully predicts pimples the next morning for everyone who's been dipping into the holiday chocolate all day. The Food and Drug Administration (FDA) announces that birth control pills can be effective at controlling acne. What a coincidence, cracks comic Conan O'Brien, reporting the news on his late-night show. "Because acne can be effective at controlling pregnancy!"

On one hand, it's hard to object to the jokes. Why shouldn't acne be fair game for humorists? After all, it's not fatal. Many women simply break out with just a pimple or two once a month—a significant annoyance, perhaps, but hardly a medical crisis.

Even extremely serious acne is not a truly grave disease. Although it is a legitimate medical disorder, in that it represents something amiss with an organ (the skin), it is neither life-threatening nor genuinely debilitating. It is not contagious. Even among skin afflictions, it barely makes the grade in terms of physical distress. It rarely itches or hurts. Nor does it, as do some more severe skin disorders, curtail the movement of a person's limbs, hamper sensation, or lay the body open to massive infection.

Well aware of all this, many women are embarrassed that acne bothers them as much as it does. They feel that they should be able to take it lightly. Rise above it. Laugh it off. "Sometimes I see someone in a wheelchair, and I feel so guilty," said Katherine, a forty-two-year-old newspaper executive, who in her mid-thirties underwent a devastating bout of adult-onset acne that left her with serious scarring. "I think to myself, my God, it's only your skin. Get over it. It's not cancer."

True. But that doesn't mean it's not serious. Women who open up about severe acne will tell you that it has permeated every aspect of their lives, blighting family, work, and social relationships. Even moderate acne can be emotionally debilitating.

"My view is that counting pimples doesn't tell you how serious the disease is," declares Dr. Albert Kligman. "Every *month* you get two pimples? In a visible place, two pimples is a big problem, and I take it seriously."

"Everyone feels the effects emotionally," adds Wexler. "Women who have acne come in here crying. They don't look you in the eye. They look at the floor. They wear turtlenecks. They wear bangs. They wear their hair in their faces. They all wear excessive amounts of makeup. Especially on the eyes, to detract from the skin. It looks as if they've thrown their makeup in the air and didn't see where it landed. Because they'll just do anything to draw attention away from their faces."

IT DOESN'T HAVE TO BE THAT WAY

Acne's capacity to inflict that kind of distress, or to affect anyone's life to the extent that it so often does, is totally out of proportion to its importance as a disease. As a leading dermatology textbook puts it: "Acne is not life-threatening, but rather life-spoiling."

But it doesn't have to be.

If you have acne, it is because your skin happens to behave that way. Just like a lot of other women's. It is prone to—or biologically programmed to—break out under certain conditions, whatever those may be in your particular case.

It's not your fault. It's not something you did. It's not something you ate. It's not something that should embarrass you. It's not something you shouldn't talk about. It's not something to be ashamed of. It shouldn't stop you from doing anything you want to do.

Acne shouldn't have that power. And the more you learn about it, the less it will.

Chapter Three

———◦———

Understanding Acne

ALTHOUGH IT OFTEN SEEMS THAT WAY, acne doesn't just pop up overnight. By the time you see an obvious blemish—whether it is a whitehead, a blackhead, or an inflamed red pimple—it is already many weeks old, the product of a complex series of events that has been taking place deep inside your skin, unseen, unfelt, and largely unaffected by anything you've done on the surface.

(Yes, I know. You try out a new makeup, and the next morning, you wake up with a crop of brand-new pimples. But, the fact is, either those pimples are not really brand new—their infant selves have been lurking in your skin for weeks—or what you see is not real acne, but rather an irritant reaction that just *looks* like acne; see Chapter 4.)

Real acne—*acne vulgaris*, as it is properly known—is born in a tiny world all its own called the "pilosebaceous unit," more popularly known as the hair follicle. In the introduction to their classic textbook *Acne and Rosacea*, pioneering acne researchers Dr. Gerd Plewig, professor and chairman of the department of dermatology at the University of Munich, and Dr. Albert Kligman, the University of Pennsylvania's retired chair of dermatology, somewhat fancifully suggest that the unseen pilosebaceous unit is a kind of "theater," a minute arena in which the "unusual drama" of acne formation unfolds.

It takes a careful viewing of this drama to appreciate just what is happening to your skin when it breaks out.

SETTING THE STAGE

The pilosebaceous unit consists of the hair follicle itself (the channel through which a hair grows) and an attached sebaceous gland, which produces the skin oil, sebum.

There are three types of hair follicle. Those known as vellus follicles are the tiniest and most numerous; they bear the downy wisps that make up the fine fuzz covering much of our bodies. Terminal follicles are much larger; they produce thick, visible hairs, including those that grow from our scalps. Acne rarely appears in either vellus or terminal follicles, because in both, the hairs are about the same diameter as the channels through which they grow. The snug fit leaves little room for pimple-causing debris to accumulate, and sebum is efficiently wicked to the surface, keeping the follicle free of oil buildup.

Things are very different in the third type of follicle, the sebaceous follicle, which is where acne usually occurs. Sebaceous follicles are concentrated on the face, neck, shoulders, upper chest, and back. They are largest and most numerous on the face, which is why acne is more common on the face than on any other part of the body.

Sebaceous follicles seem almost fiendishly well designed to produce acne blemishes. They have huge oil glands, wide follicular channels, and generous openings to the skin. (These are the pores you see when you peer closely at yourself in a mirror.) But instead of an appropriate-sized hair, the sebaceous follicle produces a frail, all-but-invisible strand that wafts loosely in the capacious channel. This leaves ample room for the series of mischief-making events that conspire to create acne.

OIL PRODUCTION

One key event is the surge of sebum that typically occurs in puberty when youngsters start to produce the hormones known as androgens. In terms of acne, the most significant androgen is testosterone, which originates in the testes in men, in the ovaries in women, and in the adrenal glands of both. Testosterone circulates via the bloodstream to reach the hair follicles, where an enzyme manufactured in the skin transforms it into a chemical called dihydrotestosterone—DHT for short. DHT signals the sebaceous glands to start producing sebum.

People who are prone to acne tend to produce higher-than-average amounts of sebum. This gives them oily skin—seborrhea, as it is called. Seborrhea has no direct link with what you eat; the fats and oil in your diet are broken down by the digestive system, and there is no pathway from there to the skin.

Nor is sebum production influenced by anything you apply to your skin. No matter how dry or tight they may make your face feel, astringent soaps, lotions, or cosmetics that mop up oil on the skin's surface cannot retard sebum output. Nor, contrary to popular belief, do they stimulate the sebaceous glands to overcompensate by stepping up oil production to lubricate the dried-out surface. Sebum output is strictly under the domination of hormones that are indifferent to cleansers, toners, and other topical oil-control treatments.

The connection between hormones and sebum does not necessarily mean that if you have excess oil on your face, your body is producing an overabundance of testosterone, or that your skin boasts an excess of follicle-stimulating DHT. It is instead, typically, a sign that your sebaceous follicles are supersensitive to these hormones and that they overreact to them, sending out the gush of shine-creating oil that is the most common feature of acne-prone skin.

"BLOCKED PORES"

Although sebum-rich sebaceous follicles provide the setting for acne, oily skin alone does not guarantee that you will break out. In fact, as you get older, your sebum production may decline, giving you skin that actually feels fairly dry—although you will still have all the oil you need to contribute to breakouts.

At any age, the main event in acne is what is known as "comedogenesis," or the production of comedones. (The singular form is "comedo.") Comedones are what we think of as blocked pores, although the term is somewhat misleading.

The word *pore* simply means "opening." There are two kinds of pore on your face: the minute apertures to hair follicles (including the sebaceous follicles, where acne occurs) and the minuscule openings to tiny sweat glands. The distinction is important because sweat glands and sweat production are not directly linked to acne. That is why you cannot, either by gentle steaming in a spa or vigorous exercise in the gym, sweat your skin free of acne-causing blockages (or, for that matter, "impurities" or "toxins"). The sweat comes from a different gland and emerges onto the skin through a totally separate pore.

The pores that count when it comes to acne are those leading down into the sebaceous follicles. Comedones are created below these openings, deep inside the follicular channel.

The popular conception of a comedo—that of a plug blocking the pore like the cork in the neck of a wine bottle—is faulty. Comedones do not typically start with surface blockages that trap oil or debris inside follicles. This is why abrasive scrubs, special cleansers, and other skin-care products that purport to "uncap" blackheads, or "unplug" pores, generally have little significant impact on acne. Rather, the blockages that lead to acne form deep inside follicles and fill them entirely. (Instead of picturing a bottle with a cork in it, try envisioning a full bottle with its contents frozen solid.)

Comedones occur when something goes awry with the skin cells that line the follicular channel. These cells are an extension of the top layer of the skin (the epidermis), which folds in and out of the follicles. As part of the normal process of skin renewal, the multilayered epidermis continuously replaces itself from the bottom up, forming a new layer of cells every few hours. New epidermal cells relentlessly push older ones up toward the surface, where eventually they are rubbed off by clothing or bedsheets, or drift unseen into the air.

Humans discard their redundant skin cells—called keratinocytes because they are made of a protein called keratin—at a prodigious rate, more than a million each hour. (In a typical household, the chief constituent of house dust, as well as the fodder for allergy-provoking dust mites, are the skin cells shed each day by the human inhabitants.) The same boundless production also occurs inside each sebaceous follicle, which, if all goes according to plan, continually expels its keratinocytes onto the surface in the normal flow of sebum.

But the process malfunctions in some follicles. Two things happen. First of all, the follicle actually steps up production of keratinocytes. No one knows precisely why or how it happens, but acne-prone follicles produce keratinocytes at a rate of about four times that of normal follicles. This creates a huge amount of cellular debris. Moreover, the excess cells, due to some chemical mechanism that medical researchers also still cannot fully explain, stick together, as if cemented, preventing them from leaving the follicle. They are, in other words, "retained." Thus, the process is sometimes called "retention hyperkeratosis" and eventually, it produces what is known as a "microcomedo"—a collection of gummed-together cells incorporated into a matrix of waxy sebum.

TINY TIME BOMBS OF ACNE

You cannot easily see or feel a microcomedo, but if you have acne, or acne-prone skin, your skin is full of them. They are what doctors call the "precursor lesions" of acne. Every manifestation of true acne, whether it is a blackhead or whitehead, a small red bump or a massive pustule, starts out as one of these little dermatological land mines.

Some microcomedones never grow past infancy. They sit in their follicles, oil flows around them and to the surface, and eventually the skin expels them. But, in some follicles (no one knows why it happens in some follicles and not others), microcomedones evolve. Over time, as cells accumulate, sebum collects, and growing hairs become encoiled and trapped inside, the little kernels get bigger and bigger. After about six to eight weeks, they grow sufficiently to make their presence known as closed comedones—small bumps you can see and feel, especially if you stretch your skin taut. If there are enough of these in any one area, that part of your skin may feel a little rough or grainy to the touch.

At this point, a closed comedo may proceed to mature into an open comedo, otherwise known as a blackhead. As the comedo continues to grow, it expands its girth from top to bottom, pressing the pore open at the surface. The skin pigment melanin, which is present in all epidermal cells, accumulates at the top and turns the visible top portion dark brown or black. (The dark color is not caused by dirt of any kind.)

Blackheads are relatively harmless skin lesions. They may look unattractive, but they almost never turn into the red pimples that are so much more objectionable in appearance and that can leave permanent scars. Blackheads typically grow to a certain size—anywhere from 2 to 5 millimeters (roughly pinhead to pencil-lead size). They may then remain in place for months or even years, without seeming to change. Cell production inside the follicle slows to a crawl, and the sebaceous glands effectively waste away, all but ceasing to excrete oil. Essentially, the mature blackhead just sits there, even though imperceptibly, it will continue to undergo glacial change as bacterial enzymes inside it dissolve old keratinocytes, and new keratinocytes slowly accumulate around the perimeter.

A whitehead is a closed comedo that takes an alternate path. Instead of pressing open the pore as it grows, the comedo expands just beneath the pore, which stays constricted, as if drawn tight by a purse string. The comedo enlarges into a palpable knot, typically with a tiny white tip at the surface.

Some whiteheads behave much like blackheads. They reach a certain size (rarely much more than 2 millimeters) and then stay put. This is what happens to people who have what is known as noninflammatory acne; they rarely get red pimples, but instead wind up with a mixture of open and closed comedones.

Noninflammatory acne runs the gamut from seemingly flawless complexions barely marred by a few tiny whiteheads, to skin the texture of coarse sandpaper, densely dotted with obvious blackheads, whiteheads, or a combination of both. Technically, it's all acne, even if it's not the obvious red bumps we think of when we hear the term.

Those bumps—pimples, zits, spots, papules, pustules, nodules, cysts—are all part of the widely variable repertoire of what is known as inflammatory acne.

BACTERIAL BUILDUP AND INFLAMMA'

Doctors still do not fully understand inflammatory acne. And the course of a visibly inflamed pimple may vary greatly from one person to another—or from one lesion to another on the same person. But in most cases, there is one obvious culprit: a tough, rod-shaped bacterium called *Propionibacterium acnes*—*P. acnes* for short. *P. acnes* are what is known as anaerobes, which means that they thrive in places where there is no oxygen. And they feed on sebum, making the constricted, oil-rich sebaceous follicles an ideal environment for them. (It is extremely useful to remember that *P. acnes* are not typically found *on* the skin, exposed to deadly air. Rather, they are deep *in* the skin. With few exceptions, the disinfectant ingredients found in most anti-bacterial facial products have little impact on them at all because these topical ingredients kill only surface organisms, leaving the *P. acnes* inside their follicular chambers unaffected.)

In the airless confines of closed comedones, *P. acnes* quickly multiply into teeming colonies. As these communities grow, they excrete a variety of toxic chemicals that damage the lining of the follicle. Among these are fatty acids (which contribute to the formation of comedones) and other irritating substances, called chemotactic factors, that seep through the follicle walls and attract the attention of the body's immune system. Neutrophils (white blood cells) respond by congregating in the area and insinuating themselves through the permeable follicular wall into the follicle to seek out and destroy the bacteria. This is the point at which you may start to sense or feel something—a little tenderness, perhaps a slight elevation under the skin.

Contrary to the common understanding of pimple formation, in which a blocked follicle steadily inflates with accumulating oil and other material until it bursts like a balloon to spew its contents into the skin and give you a red zit, follicles do not typically break under pressure. (That is, not unless you apply the pressure yourself, by aggressive squeezing.) Instead, as the *P. acnes*–seeking neutrophils find their bacterial targets in the follicle, they release protein-dissolving enzymes that destroy some part of the follicular wall, creating a rupture.

This can (and frequently does) happen when comedones are still in their microscopic infancy—long before you see an obvious blockage or perceive any substantial buildup of sebum or other material. In fact, many people (in particular women with adult acne) who suffer from severe inflammatory acne, with multiple angry red bumps and nodules, never get visible whiteheads or blackheads at all. This may be because they have unusually fragile follicles that virtually disintegrate at the microcomedo stage, succumbing readily to the corrosive chain of events set off by the presence of *P. acnes*. Or their skin's immune response may be so exquisitely tuned that the presence of the tiny microcomedo incites an explosive inflammatory reaction at the very earliest stages.

What happens next is determined by a number of factors, including the size and location of the rupture, the amount of material that escapes through it, and, most crucial of all, the unique immune responses of your own skin.

PAPULES, PUSTULES, CYSTS— AND DREADED "CHIN ACNE"

Sometimes, when a follicle breaks, the body quickly repairs the breach, and the tender spot you feared was sure to turn into a major pimple simply calms down and goes away. Sometimes, it will proceed to become a papule, a red, raised spot without a visible head. (The redness comes from densely packed networks of microscopic blood vessels that spring up to serve as a kind of vascular railroad for neutrophils and other substances; the swelling is caused by the accumulation of lymph and other fluids.)

Individual follicles can go through this rupture-and-repair scenario repeatedly. This is what, in some women, causes a succession of tender bumps that periodically come and go, never quite coming to a head and turning into what we think of as full-fledged pimples.

But if the body does not manage to repair the break quickly, the contents of the follicle—sebum, bits of hair, bacteria, horny skin cells—all spill into the surrounding tissue. Armies of neutrophils rush to the area to gobble up, isolate, and expel the invading materials. In the process they release more protein-dissolving enzymes that destroy more of the follicle wall, as well as surrounding tissues in the skin's fibrous middle layer, the dermis.

If this activity takes place fairly near the surface, you will see the result within about seventy-two hours as a pustule, a white or yellow-capped acne lesion filled with pus, which contains spent white blood cells, bacteria, and other debris. Typically, the roof of the pustule eventually bursts and the pus escapes, carrying with it all or most of the horny remnants of the comedo. Sometimes this marks the end of activity in that follicle, and it never again produces another pimple. In other cases, bits of material are left behind to eventually seed the growth of a successor comedo—sometimes called a secondary comedo. This is what causes that phenomenon in which individual pimples seem to come back over and over again in the very same locations. (The material that leaks or bursts onto the skin does not in itself lead to new breakouts.)

The larger lesions, known as nodules or cysts, usually begin with more extensive follicular ruptures much deeper in the skin and can take literally months to heal. Sometimes, two or more adjoining follicles become involved simultaneously and link up to form a monster zit. There is no easy path to the surface, so the inflammation spreads beneath the surface and more dermal tissue is destroyed. When the nodule eventually does come to a head and open, bits of horny material and other debris are inevitably left behind, prolonging the inflammation and often seeding new secondary comedones. Again, you may have a large pimple, or a colony of them, that seems to rise and fall continuously at the same location.

Persistent secondary comedones—whether small papules or monster cysts—are extremely common in women with acne, frequently found on the chin or along the jawline, and they can be very difficult to eliminate. "These are really feared lesions, because they are so asymmetrical that they do not have a chance to resolve spontaneously or heal through natural mechanisms," explains Dr. Gerd Plewig. "They are held deep in the skin, stuff cannot come out, they stay inflamed, and go on and on."

ACNE SCARRING

Ironically (because the inflammatory process, after all, is part of the body's own defense mechanism), inflammatory acne is enormously destructive. It turns your face into a battlefield whose terrain is constantly being torn up, marked, and altered.

Long after an individual pimple heals, the red spot (called a macule) that it leaves behind may linger, as the tiny blood vessels that sprang up in that area slowly wither away. Large nodules and cysts leave permanent depressions, ranging from shallow dimples to sharply delineated pits, showing where sections of the fibrous collagen network in the dermis have been destroyed. In some cases, the skin responds to its injuries by manufacturing extra collagen to effect a repair; the super-fluous tissue builds up on the skin as a raised scar.

Hidden follicular ruptures that heal before ever appearing on the exterior bequeath internal scars, sometimes evident on the surface as subtle skin irregularities. Even the most seem-ingly insignificant and superficial pimples leave their imprint, even if they do not produce an obvious defect. Healed follicles never return to their precise original size and shape; the expe-rience of harboring an inflamed comedo always permanently distorts the channel to some extent. You may not be able see these tiny anomalies with the naked eye, but over time, as they accumulate, they contribute to the coarse, irregular-appearing texture that characterizes acne-prone skin.

ACNE IN SKIN OF COLOR

Acne occurs in the same manner and at about the same rate in women of color as in Caucasians. But breakouts on skin of color can have even more distressing long-term consequences. The most common are dark spots that remain long after the original blemishes have healed. These marks, which doctors call hyper-pigmented macules, are the result of dark skin's tendency to re-spond to injury by turning perceptibly darker—a phenomenon known as post-inflammatory hyperpigmentation.

All humans owe their skin color to the pigment melanin, a chemical compound created by specialized cells called melanocytes. Melanin is the body's first line of defense against destructive sunlight, functioning as a filter against ultraviolet rays. Melanin may also act in some way to ward off certain toxins and to counteract the damaging effect of free oxygen radicals. Thus, any assault on the skin—particularly any injury that causes the skin to become inflamed—can trigger melanocytes to jump into action and step up their production of protective melanin. (This is what produces a suntan, the most familiar example of post-inflammatory hyperpigmentation; it is the skin's response to the injury inflicted by ultraviolet light.) An acne lesion—which is a small spot of intense inflammation—can have a similar effect, and the accumulation of melanin will show up as a brown discoloration.

Physicians still do not fully understand why it happens, but the melanocytes in dark skin tend to respond much more rapidly and efficiently to injury than do melanocytes in pale skin. "People with skin of color have *very* reactive melanocytes," says Dr. Susan Taylor, director of the Skin of Color Center at New York's St. Luke's–Roosevelt Hospital Center. "With inflammation they are going to produce more melanin." The result for dark-skinned acne patients is that inflamed pimples frequently leave discolorations that may last for months, or even years, after the original lesion has disappeared.

"My typical acne patients of color, including Asians and light-skinned African Americans and Hispanics, tend to be a lot less bothered by acne pimples than they are by these dark marks the pimples leave," says Taylor. "They come in and say, 'How do I get rid of these spots!' Not the pimple or the papule, but the spots. It's a significant problem."

Another potential problem for dark skin is that its fibroblasts, the cells in the dermis that produce collagen, have a somewhat greater tendency than those in Caucasian skin to repair an injury by producing excess new collagen. If that happens, as an inflamed acne lesion heals, the result will be a raised scar (what doctors call a hypertrophic scar), or even a keloid, a raised scar that spreads out over the skin, growing well beyond the boundaries of the original blemish.

ACNE "BURNOUT" AND OTHER MYSTERIES

In anyone with acne, of whatever age, sex, or skin type, only some sebaceous follicles ever break out at any one time. Somehow, certain follicles seem fated to produce acne at some point in their lives; others do not. No one knows why. It is a puzzle that still baffles doctors who have spent decades studying acne.

"To me, one of the most incredible mysteries is, how come only some follicles are involved at any one time," says Albert Kligman. "You've got thousands of sebaceous follicles on your face—a hell of a lot. But maybe you've only got ten or fifteen or twenty comedones. Here's one follicle with a comedo, and right next door, there's one that's normal. Why is that? Whatever it is, we simply don't know."

"I think there is a rhythm to the follicles," comments Plewig. "Some are quiescent, others become more active. This explains the coming and going of acne. But the biological controls are still a mystery."

A related mystery is the age-related pattern in which breakouts typically appear. Acne in young people commonly occurs in the middle of the face, first showing up on the nose, then moving up on to the forehead. As a person gets a little older, the blemishes tend to migrate outward, over the cheeks. Finally, they work their way down onto the chin, along the jawline, and sometimes down onto the neck. Adult women with acne often wind up with just a few persistent pimples that show up only on the chin or jaw.

In most cases, acne eventually disappears. This is what doctors call acne burnout—or, simply, "outgrowing it." By their early to mid-twenties, most men and women who had acne as teens are no longer breaking out. "For some reason the follicles

are no longer capable of developing comedones," says Kligman. "And we don't know the reason for that either."

Nor do doctors know why those women (and some men)
whose follicles clearly *are* still capable of developing comedones continue to break out well past their twenties. Any
more than they understand why some people get acne in the
first place, and others do not, and why it varies so in severity.
Everyone who reaches puberty produces sebum and harbors
P. acnes bacteria. Yet only some people get acne. Of those, only
some get inflamed pimples. Again, it is a mystery.

"The events in each person and in each follicle are completely unpredictable," says Kligman. "In some people you'll
see pimples come up and disappear in two days. In others
you'll see pimples that look absolutely the same, and they stay
there for two weeks. I don't understand it. A lot of people
have pustules all over, and you'll never see a scar. Similar people get one pimple and the damn thing leaves a scar. I don't
know why that happens either. No one does."

THINGS THAT AREN'T ACNE

Because acne is so common, it is very easy to assume that
every time you see a crop of what look like pimples, you have,
indeed, got acne. Doctors once thought so, too, lumping a
commodious medical grab bag of pimply, pustular-appearing
skin disorders into the same convenient category. But as dermatologists have learned more about the multiple factors that
cause acne, they have refined the ways in which it is classified.

Today, common acne—*acne vulgaris*—is defined as a disease that starts with a microcomedo. This definition encom-
passes a wide range of variants and subtypes, from very mild
collections of small comedones to the most virulent forms of

inflammatory acne. On the other hand, a number of other skin disorders that look very much like acne and were once regarded as acne variants are now classified instead as "acneiform eruptions." In an acneiform eruption, there is no comedo; what doctors call the primary lesion is the inflamed papule or pustule itself.

Many skin conditions can produce these acne-like pimples. Some are very rare, and only a dermatologist with experience in arcane skin diseases can correctly diagnose them. Others are quite common, among them acne rosacea, sometimes misleadingly called "adult acne," and various forms of folliculitis, which is an inflammation of the hair follicle, typically caused by irritation, chemicals, or a bacterial or fungal infection. For example, a common acne-like complaint called perioral dermatitis (tiny, irritated, red bumps that crop up around the mouth) is a form of folliculitis. So, too, are many of the pimple-like eruptions brought on by the ingredients in cosmetics or skin-care products.

Milia, another common skin eruption, is caused by an accumulation of horny material in tiny sweat gland ducts; the small white or yellowish bumps are sometimes confused with the whiteheads seen in noninflammatory acne.

Chapter Four

◦

"Will It Make Me Break Out?"

LIVE WITH ACNE FOR ANY NUMBER OF YEARS and you inevitably develop a little censor in your head, a small inner voice, always ready to chime in with the same worrisome question: "Will it make me break out?"

"If I put on that makeup, will it make me break out?" "I've got a job interview next week. Will I break out?" "If I take this pill, will I break out?" "I'm getting married next month. . . . Oh, God! I'll definitely break out!" "If I eat this . . ." "If I wear that . . ." "If I do whatever . . ."

Will I break out?

If you have acne-prone skin, all too often the answer is yes. Your sebaceous follicles are like little dermatological Achilles heels—biological weak links that may succumb at any time to any number of internal or external influences to give you acne. Or to make the acne you already have even worse.

In women, acne is frequently triggered by the natural hormonal shifts that govern our reproductive lives. Ovulation, menstruation, pregnancy, nursing a baby, or going through menopause can all affect the hormones that stimulate sebaceous glands, and thus bring on or worsen acne. Or, conversely and mysteriously, improve it or make it go away (see Chapter 8). And although researchers have begun only recently to seriously investigate the link between acne and the mind, it has long appeared clear to many women and their doctors that stress is also a potent factor in instigating and aggravating breakouts (see Chapter 10).

But sebaceous follicles and the hormones that control them are also vulnerable to a host of other acne-aggravating influences that, yes indeed, may well make you break out.

COSMETICS AND SKIN-CARE PRODUCTS

For decades, dermatologists suspected that postadolescent acne in women was caused by the cosmetics they used on their faces. In fact, *acne cosmetica*, as acne brought on by cosmetics is called, was widely believed to be the reason that so many more grown women than grown men got acne.

Doctors now know that genetic predisposition and hormonal influences play a far more significant role than any cosmetic or skin-care product in determining who gets acne and who doesn't. Moreover, the cosmetic products found in stores today are much less likely than those of a generation ago to contain genuinely comedogenic substances—that is, agents that block or occlude normal follicles and affect them in such a way that comedones develop and eventually evolve into genuine acne (i.e., *acne vulgaris*, or comedonal acne).

"There used to be many more offensive ingredients in cosmetics," notes Dr. Alan Shalita, chairman of the department of dermatology at the State University of New York, and a leading acne researcher. "Some of those old creams and pomades would give anyone acne. Today, true cosmetic acne is unusual because the companies, for the most part, have done a very good job of removing most of the offensive ingredients."

However, even if a given cosmetic may not cause true

comedonal acne, it may still make you break out. This can be substantiated by any acne-prone woman who has had the unhappy experience of trying out a new makeup and waking up the next morning (or a couple of days later) with a face full of angry red pimples. Typically, these are not true acne lesions, but acneiform eruptions—acne-like breakouts in which there are no comedones.

"The breakouts that appear overnight from acnegenic products are not *acne cosmetica*," emphasizes Munich's Dr. Gerd Plewig. "Comedones do not come overnight. Irritation comes overnight, and then you have what is known as chemical folliculitis."

Chemical folliculitis, which is an irritated, inflamed follicle induced by some agent applied to the skin, is sort of a good-news, bad-news situation for those prone to acne. On the one hand, it's not true acne—which, of course, is good news. And because it occurs so quickly, you will probably immediately know—or at least suspect—what caused it. That's good, too, because you can stop using that particular product, and your grateful skin will probably respond by clearing itself up within a week or two. (If it does not, a dermatologist can prescribe antibiotics or other appropriate treatment.)

The bad news is that chemical irritation can substantially aggravate any acne you already have, turning small, inconspicuous pimples or comedones into big, red, obvious ones. Moreover, many irritating substances, while not truly comedogenic in the strict sense of the word, can lead to comedonal acne in acne-prone skin. "Stimulation through chemical folliculitis can start the process," warns Plewig. "If you see chemical folliculitis—if you have irritation—you may be turning on that follicle, and it can eventually develop a comedo."

Low-grade inflammation may also directly stimulate sebum production. And irritation has also been shown to increase the size of the sebaceous glands in both humans and in laboratory mice.

This is why many dermatologists are increasingly likely to regard irritating substances in cosmetics as being as much of a problem for acne-prone women as the classic occlusive, comedogenic ingredients they have always told us to avoid. Ironically, many of these irritating substances can be found in the very products acne patients have traditionally used to make their acne better. Alcohol, menthol, peppermint, eucalyptus, camphor, lemon, grapefruit, and similar ingredients, which have long been used in acne preparations to impart a brisk, bracing, presumably antiseptic sensation, can all be extremely irritating and may result in angry red breakouts in acne-prone skin.

COSMETICS AND TRUE COMEDOGENICITY

True *acne cosmetica*, which develops over time, is unlikely to be red and inflamed. "Cosmetics don't give you cysts or nodules," says dermatologist Marianne O'Donoghue. "What you get from cosmetics will be that muddy complexion with lots of little bumps."

The lesions typically show up as small, closely packed whiteheads appearing in the same pattern in which you've applied the offending product. For example, the bumps will be clustered around your lips if they are caused by a comedogenic substance in your lipstick or lip balm (doctors sometimes call this "Chapstick acne"). Acne will appear on your cheekbone if it comes from an ingredient in a bronzer or blusher; or it will crop up along your hairline from a comedogenic hair product. So-called "pomade acne" is a variation of *acne cosmetica* seen commonly among African Americans. It appears on the forehead or around the temples, caused by

heavy hair-conditioning treatments and scalp oils used to protect the hair.

Cocoa butter is another common acne promoter for black
women, warns Washington, D.C., dermatologist Cheryl Burgess.
"It's so common in the African American community. My grand-
mother used it on everything: burns, skinned knees, ashy skin,
you name it. But it is very comedogenic; just terrible for acne-
prone skin."

Today, both doctors and cosmetic manufacturers frequently make a distinction between a given product's comedogenic potential (its tendency to form comedones) and its
acnegenic or pustulogenic potential—that is, its tendency to
generate inflamed bumps or pustules.

That is why some cosmetic products may be labeled "non-
comedogenic" and others "non-acnegenic"—or sometimes
both. Neither of the terms has any official or legal meaning
(they're not sanctioned by the FDA or any other regulatory
body), but "non-comedogenic" is generally accepted to mean
that a product does not contain ingredients that have been
tested and proven to generate comedones. (Ingredients used to
be tested for comedogenicity on rabbits' ears; today, they are
patch-tested on women's backs.) "Non-acnegenic" typically
means that the finished product has been used for a number of
weeks by women volunteers, and that it did not cause breakouts—either acneiform eruptions or comedonal acne.

Does this mean that if you use a product labeled non-
comedogenic or non-acnegenic, you won't break out? You
probably already know the answer to that one. Of course not.
There is no way to predict with absolute certainty how any
one woman will react to the specific combination of ingredients in any given product. "When we say a product is non-
comedogenic, we mean that for the majority of women, the
ingredients in that product will not cause comedones,"

explains O'Donoghue. "But there is no such thing as a product being absolutely non-comedogenic or non-acnegenic. It only means that most people can put it on and not get blackheads or pimples."

Trying to identify potentially troublesome cosmetics by perusing labels for comedogenic or acnegenic ingredients is not only frustrating and incredibly confusing, it is also largely futile. Any product's potential for causing breakouts is likely to lie more in the manner in which it is formulated than in any of its individual parts. In other words, an ingredient that might give you a pimple in one product can be totally inoffensive when mixed into another.

Seeking out and sticking with non-comedogenic- or non-acnegenic-labeled products made by reputable cosmetic companies (who test their products and can back up their claims with the test results) is one of your best bets for remaining breakout-free from skin products. Otherwise, it is—alas—largely a matter of trial and error, avoiding extremely thick, creamy, or oil-rich products in favor or those formulated as lightweight lotions, gels, or serums.

And quickly abandoning any product that irritates or reddens your skin.

CHEMICAL AND OCCUPATIONAL ACNE

Chemical acne (sometimes called "occupational acne") is caused by exposure to comedogenic or acnegenic industrial chemicals. It is most often found among industrial workers who are in regular contact with the offending chemicals, although others may sometimes be exposed to the same chemicals in contaminated wastes or consumer products. For example, hobbyists such as gardeners, sailors, or do-it-yourselfers who work on their own automobiles or home construction projects will sometimes come into contact with comedogenic industrial agents.

Occupational acne falls into three general categories: oil acne, which is caused by exposure to petroleum products such as machine oil and cutting oils (particularly when oil-soaked clothing clings for hours on end to the skin); coal-tar acne, which comes from coal tar derivatives, including pitch and creosote; and choracne, a virulent and potentially scar-ring form of acne that shows up three to four weeks after the skin has been exposed to chemicals known as halogenated aromatic compounds. Choracne is a potential hazard for workers in chemical manufacturing plants, laboratories, or waste-handling facilities, but the compounds may also be found in some insecticides, pesticides, herbicides, or wood preservatives.

PRESCRIPTION DRUGS

A number of prescription drugs taken for various medical con-ditions can either bring on acne or aggravate existing break-outs. Some drugs are excreted through the sebaceous follicles, thus directly stimulating breakouts; others affect acne by influencing the hormones that control the sebaceous glands.

Among these potential acne aggravators are some of the more commonly prescribed central nervous system medica-tions, including barbiturates, antiseizure medicines (for exam-ple, Dilantin, which is used to treat epilepsy), and psychotropic medicines such as lithium. "Every single patient I've ever seen on lithium has terrible acne," notes dermatologist Laurie Polis. "And if you don't know she's taking it, you can treat and treat and treat the acne, and never get anywhere."

Other potential acne aggravators include isoniazid, a drug used to treat tuberculosis, and gonadotropins (drugs that are prescribed for some pituitary disorders and that can aggravate acne by stimulating the production of testosterone).

If you have any of these conditions, it is important to discuss your medication both with your dermatologist and with the specialist who prescribed the drug to see if less skin-damaging alternatives can be found.

STEROIDS

By far the most common acne-stimulating drugs are the steroids, which are close chemical cousins of androgens and can have similar effects on the skin. The anabolic (i.e., muscle-building) steroids used by some athletes (legally, to rehabilitate injuries; illegally, to bulk up and boost performance) are well known to bodybuilders as a cause of acne. A less well-recognized threat to your skin is the popular hormonal supplement DHEA, which is sold in health food stores as an antiaging agent.

DHEA is an androgen that occurs naturally in your body, produced by the adrenal glands. The body converts it, as needed, into estrogen and testosterone. Levels of natural DHEA begin to drop off in your thirties; the dietary supplement (derived from wild yams) is promoted as a near-miraculous substitute that supposedly will boost your libido, strengthen your immune system, and add years to your life—while at the same time reducing wrinkles and improving the overall appearance of your skin.

But the long-term health effects of supplemental DHEA (which is not regulated by the FDA) are unknown, causing endocrinologists to characterize it as a risky gamble. In women, the short-term, steroidal side effects, which may appear within a few months (and can include weight gain, excess facial and body hair, male pattern baldness, as well as pimples), have led some dermatologists to call DHEA the "acne supplement."

Overuse, or the improper use, of the topical corticosteroids to treat many inflammatory skin conditions can also wreak acne havoc, warns Polis. "Fluorinated steroids—which are strong steroids used for conditions like psoriasis—should almost never be used on the face, because if even a little bit rolls on nonaffected areas, it can cause acne."

Dr. Susan Taylor of New York's Skin of Color Center also warns against the strong steroid creams used by some African American women as skin-bleaching agents. These can backfire both by overlightening the skin and by triggering acne.

A nightmarish vicious circle may also arise if a woman tries to use a topical steroid to treat inflamed red pimples. "This happens a lot," says Polis. "A woman will get a steroid cream from a primary care doctor who doesn't recognize all the different types of acne. Or maybe a dermatologist who means well will give her a steroid to use for just a few days to calm things down. Or she'll just borrow her friend's anti-inflammation cream. Wherever she gets it, when she uses it, she'll see an immediate improvement in her acne, because the steroid makes the redness less red. So she keeps using it. The steroid, meanwhile, is thinning the skin, plugging the follicles, stimulating sebaceous secretion, promoting bacterial growth, and doing every possible thing to create folliculitis and an acne flare. Two weeks later, the acne gets worse. And she—understandably— thinks, 'Oh, my face is worse. I'd better use more of this medicine because it helps me.' And the whole tailspin begins."

SUN EXPOSURE

Sunlight can have both positive and negative effects on acne. On the one hand, sun exposure works to suppress the growth of acne-aggravating *P. acnes* bacteria; sunlight in the narrow, 410 to 420 nanometer wavelength range (or violet-blue range) is so efficient at killing *P. acnes* that the FDA recently approved a lamp that emits that type of light as an acne treatment (page 87). The sun's ultraviolet light waves also depress the immune system, which may lead to some improvement in acne by retarding the movement of white blood cells and reducing inflammation. And, of course, women with acne like to sunbathe for the same reason that women with dimpled thighs do: A good tan camouflages bumpy imperfections, whether it's pimples or cellulite.

But the drawbacks of sun exposure far outweigh any potential advantages. Ultraviolet rays ultimately do far more harm than good by altering the DNA in skin cells, setting the stage for ugly age spots and possible skin cancers. Tanning, the skin's protective response to sun damage, also thickens the stratum corneum (the outer layer of the epidermis), adding to the load of skin cells filling your follicles and creating new comedones. And there is also evidence that sunlight may stimulate oil production: Ultraviolet radiation increases the size of sebaceous glands in lab animals.

"In my practice, the busiest time of the year for acne is October," notes Polis. "People go out in the sun in the summer; the sunlight stimulates the follicles. And a few months later, you've got more acne."

Climate

In World War II, and during the Korean and Vietnamese conflicts, some of the French, British, and American soldiers fighting in the Pacific and in Southeast Asia suffered from such horrendous acne that they had to be mustered out of their respective services. Doctors called it "tropical acne." In more recent years, Northern Europeans, on returning home from island holidays, often show up a few weeks later at their dermatologists' offices with new or dramatically worsened acne, a phenomenon that has become known as "Mallorca acne," after the popular Mediterranean vacation spot.

Tropical acne and Mallorca acne are both thought to be brought on by excessively humid air, which hydrates skin cells, and can cause or exacerbate acne by making the cells packed in comedones and in the lining of sebaceous follicles swell up from the absorbed moisture. Saunas, steam baths, and facial steamers can have a similar effect, and many dermatologists now advise acne patients to avoid them.

Alternatively, dry cold air can also make acne worse. "In dry air, you get a thick gummy sebum that can cover the pores like a sheet of wax paper on the skin," says O'Donoghue. "In temperate zones, January, February, and March are the worst months for a lot of acne patients."

Sweat, Clothing, and Pressure

In and of itself, sweat or engaging in sweat-producing activities does not usually aggravate acne. But sweat that is held against the skin by, say, a hat or headband can cause the skin cells to swell just as they do in an extremely humid environment. At the same time, the pressure of cloth against the skin prevents oil from escaping, and friction irritates the pore. This can give you a bad case of what doctors sometimes anachronistically call "hippie acne" (from the headband around the forehead).

Hippie acne is more properly known as *acne mechanica*, which is acne that is caused or aggravated by pressure and friction—typically from your hands or from clothing or sports equipment. Rubbing your skin, leaning your chin on your hand, pressing a phone receiver against your face for long periods, or even sleeping every night with your cheek pressed into the pillow in the same position can all cause comedo-impacted follicles to break down into pimples and give you *acne mechanica*. *Acne mechanica* can even be caused by excessive or overly aggressive cleansing with a washcloth or an abrasive cleanser.

PICKING AND SQUEEZING

Picking pimples is a form of *acne mechanica* that occupies a special niche of its own. It's called *acne excoriee*. Or, because it is more frequently seen in women than in men, *acne excoriee des jeunes filles*.

Acne excoriee is essentially acne combined with impetigo, a superficial skin infection (more commonly seen in children than in adults) that is caused by a strep or staph infection, explains O'Donoghue. "You get *acne excoriee* where you convert acne into staph impetigo. If you have an inflammatory acne lesion and you rub it, it's going to get bigger or it's going to break open. Once it breaks open, you can get a staph infection on top of your acne, because underneath your nails, you're loaded with staph."

"It is a huge problem," agrees Plewig. "Sometimes you have minor acne, but the patient is a bad picker and she destroys her skin. It's not the disease itself; it's the fingering of the wound."

Chapter Five

————◇————

Over-the-Counter Remedies

FOR MOST WOMEN, acne treatment begins and ends at the drugstore or the cosmetics counter. Surveys have shown that the vast majority of all acne patients—around 80 percent—never see a dermatologist. According to a 2002 *Self* magazine poll, the percentage remains about the same for grown women: Only 27 percent of the readers polled said they used prescription medicine to control their acne breakouts.

For many of those who don't see a dermatologist, the non-prescription remedies found today on the shelves of retail outlets may be all that is ever needed to clear up breakouts and keep them at bay. "Over-the-counter [OTC] acne treatments work for a lot of people," says acne expert Dr. Alan Shalita. "They don't work as fast as prescription medicine. Or as effectively. But they do work. If you've got mild acne—a few pimples, a couple of comedones—you may never have to go beyond the drugstore."

The problem, of course, is that once you're inside the drugstore—or at the department store, or browsing the Internet—you are faced with a bewildering array of cleansers, toners, lotions, masks, and other products that all promise to banish blemishes, control oil, clean pores, fight shine, or otherwise combat breakouts.

In truth, you really need only a couple.
How do you choose?

ACNE-FIGHTING INGREDIENTS: THE BASICS

The first step is to distinguish the drugs from the cosmetics. Nonprescription acne fighters fall into either one category or the other. Those saying specifically on their labels that they treat acne (a bona fide medical condition) are regulated by the U.S. Food and Drug Administration (FDA) as over-the-counter drugs. Just like nasal sprays, cough syrups, or any other nonprescription medicine, all acne treatments must contain at least one FDA-approved active ingredient for that condition, in an amount that has been proven to be safe and effective.

Surprisingly, considering the sheer number of available products, there are only four FDA-approved active ingredients for acne: benzoyl peroxide, salicylic acid, sulfur, and sulfur combined with resorcinol. So, whether it is sold at Wal-Mart, Saks Fifth Avenue, or Sephora.com, any product that bears a label promising that it treats "acne" must also include at least one of those four agents in an appropriate concentration (e.g., "Benzoyl peroxide, 2.5%" or "Resorcinol, 2%; Sulfur, 8%").

Since 2002, the FDA has also required that all over-the-counter drugs bear a standardized "Drug Facts" label clearly stating its active ingredient, its purpose (in the case of acne, it's "acne medication" or "acne treatment") and its use, e.g., "for the management of acne."

By far the two most commonly used active ingredients in OTC acne medicines today are salicylic acid and benzoyl peroxide. Acne products containing sulfur and resorcinol, which were the cornerstone ingredients of nonprescription acne treatment for decades, have become relatively scarce in recent years. Some dermatologists say these traditional agents still have a role to play in treating breakouts, but benzoyl peroxide and salicylic acid, both with a long history of use and numerous studies investigating their effects, are today's key nonprescription choices.

They are not interchangeable, but work in different, complementary ways. Benzoyl peroxide is an antibacterial agent with a peerless ability to seek out and destroy the follicle-dwelling *P. acnes* bacteria implicated in inflammatory acne. Salicylic acid is a mild exfoliant and a comedolytic ingredient, which means that it works to loosen and expel comedones and microcomedones, the time-bomb "precursor lesions" of acne. It also has anti-inflammatory qualities that help tame the redness of inflamed lesions.

Unlike many of the other antibacterial and exfoliating ingredients found in skin-care products (including many of those touted as "blemish-fighting" or "pore-cleaning" potions), both benzoyl peroxide and salicylic acid are lipid soluble, which means they will cut through oil. Thus, they can penetrate into sebaceous follicles to strike acne at its roots.

Or, at least *three* of its roots: comedo formation and inflammation, in the case of salicylic acid; bacterial activity (and, indirectly, the inflammation that results from it), in the case of benzoyl peroxide. In the face of so many skin-care products advertised and labeled as having oil-control properties, it is worth emphasizing that there are no over-the-counter treatments that affect either the output of oil-producing sebaceous glands or the hormones that govern their behavior. Agents that soak up, disperse, or otherwise "control" sebum that has made its way to the surface of your skin may help it to look and feel less greasy (see Chapter 11). They may also "dry you out," by taking water out of the skin's upper layers. But superficial oil control, no matter how effective it may be at temporarily improving your appearance, plays no role in actually preventing or alleviating blemishes.

Blemish fighters that do not contain any FDA-approved acne ingredients—or include them in less than the required concentrations—are classified as "cosmetics" rather than drugs. This is the case even if they are marketed as part of an acne-fighting regimen, or sold alongside acne-drug siblings from the same manufacturer.

Labels that seem to be using acne code-speak ("problem skin" or "blemish control") instead of forthrightly announcing that the package contains an "acne" remedy are often phrased that way because the product does not include an approved ingredient in sufficient quantity. Thus it cannot legally be called an acne medicine. (Occasionally, it's a marketing ploy. Some manufacturers, particularly those who make high-end skin-care lines, prefer to downplay the adolescent-sounding "acne" in favor of less-stigmatizing references to "pores" or "shine control"—even if the package does contain a legitimate acne medicine.)

EXTRA, ADDED INGREDIENTS

As a practical matter, companies who make OTC acne remedies typically build an individual acne product around one of the approved active ingredients, and then mix anything else they think might be beneficial (vitamins, minerals, glycolic acid, retinol, tea tree oil, herbs—whatever) into the "inactive ingredients." Many of these are drawn from the vast pharmacopoeia of alternative medicine—botanical, herbal, or other ingredients, many with a long history of traditional use (see Chapter 9).

For example, Clinique's Acne Solutions Night Treatment Gel contains 2 percent salicylic acid as the active ingredient, and also includes a half dozen other "inactive" ingredients that may or may not have an impact on your acne: sea whip, green tea extract, sucrose, and kola nut, all of which are anti-inflammatory or anti-irritant agents to combat redness; sugarcane extract and glucosamine, which are both exfoliants (that is, they can peel off a layer of skin); laminaria saccharina, a seaweed extract that may help reduce surface oil; and yeast, which can work to tame discoloration.

There is a staggering number of similar botanical, mineral, and animal-derived agents that have potential therapeutic effects, but have never been subjected to the FDA's rigorous drug-approval procedure, a process that can take decades and cost tens of millions of dollars. And there is little evidence to show how these ingredients work, or even if they work at all on acne—much less in the unique formulations and often minute quantities in which they appear in most acne products. Large cosmetic companies such as Estée Lauder (parent company of Clinique) test their products thoroughly, and they employ eminent dermatologists as consultants. But for the most part they keep the details of their research private, so it is not subject to scientific scrutiny.

On the other hand, some of the supposedly inactive agents that are added to acne or other skin-care products make good theoretical sense and may well have a genuine therapeutic effect on acne. For example, any ingredient that has anti-inflammatory or anti-irritant properties is potentially beneficial in treating acne. Or, a particular formulation may simply make a product more "cosmetically elegant," that is to say, more enticing to use and less likely to produce disagreeable side effects—important considerations when it comes to acne treatments, which must be applied consistently in order to be effective. (In other words, given two acne preparations each containing benzoyl peroxide, the light, pleasant-smelling lotion that can be worn under makeup is a lot more likely to be used every day than the thick medicinal ointment that leaves a chalky residue.)

The sensible course in choosing OTC acne products, say dermatologists, is to focus on the basics: Look first for labeled acne medications containing one of the FDA-approved active ingredients. These are the tried-and-true agents that have been subjected to extensive research and are most likely to act on your blemishes in a predictable fashion. Then feel free to make a pick based on more subjective criteria—how a product looks, feels, or smells; and whether it contains any additional ingredients that you find persuasive or appealing.

WHY YOU WANT BENZOYL PEROXIDE

If you have inflammatory acne (red pimples or papules), benzoyl peroxide is, hands down, the single most potent weapon you can get without a prescription. In fact, it's one of the most potent acne fighters period. "Benzoyl peroxide really revolutionized acne treatment, " says Chicago dermatologist Marianne O'Donoghue. "It was one of the first things we had that really worked, and it's still one of the best things we've got."

"It is *very* powerful stuff," concurs Munich's professor Gerd Plewig, who sternly maintains that, otherwise, "Good acne drugs do *not* come over the counter," and dismisses all other OTC acne ingredients as minor players—"bystanders only."

Benzoyl peroxide operates on acne by releasing oxygen into the airless confines of sebaceous follicles to kill the oxygen-phobic *P. acnes* bacteria. Benzoyl draws the peroxide into the follicle; the peroxide releases the oxygen that destroys the bacteria. It also has mild comedolytic effects: By reducing *P. acnes*, it cuts down on the comedogenic fatty acids that the bacteria produce, thus helping to loosen comedones. Benzoyl peroxide works quickly, suppressing *P. acnes* even faster than prescription antibiotics. And unlike antibiotics, benzoyl peroxide never loses its effectiveness because bacteria do not become resistant to it.

No other topical antimicrobial or antibacterial agent has been shown to precisely match these effects. "And, believe me, people have looked," says Shalita. "For example, hydrogen peroxide is not stable enough; it explodes on the surface, so it doesn't get down into the follicle. Alcohol doesn't work. Neither do the old antibacterials we used to use, like triclosan or the hexachlorophene in pHisoHex; none of them get into the follicle and do the job."

The key to getting the most out of benzoyl peroxide is to use it preventively—to kill off *P. acnes* before they get out of hand and ignite the destructive inflammatory process that gives you a pimple. This means you should apply it every day, all over the entire area of skin where you typically break out—even if your skin looks perfectly clear. If you wait until you see a red spot, and dab the lotion or cream on it, you're essentially too late. The redness is a sign that your body has already sent bacteria-battling neutrophils in, and they're busy killing off *P. acnes*—and producing those destructive inflammatory reactions. And if you dot benzoyl peroxide on a pustule, it will have even less effect. Pus is a sign of dead bacteria—an indication that the battle is all but over in that particular spot.

Curiously, many benzoyl peroxide acne medicines are either sold as spot treatments, or named in such a way that you would think they were spot treatments (Neutrogena's On-the-Spot Acne Treatment and Clinique's Acne Solutions Emergency Gel, for example). Nonetheless, emphasizes Shalita, "benzoyl peroxide is not intended to be a spot treatment. Its primary function is preventative."

Used correctly, benzoyl peroxide really can keep many common forms of acne well under control. Witness the success of Proactiv, the best-selling line of acne products in the world today, and an empire largely built on the power of benzoyl peroxide. When Proactiv was introduced in 1992, most other OTC benzoyl peroxide products contained high concentrations that many users found too irritating for daily use. Proactiv's benzoyl peroxide cleanser and treatment lotion (part of a three-step daily regimen) were formulated to mimic the cosmetically elegant feel and smell of prestige skin-care lines. Both contain benzoyl peroxide in a mild concentration (2.5 percent) that most acne sufferers can tolerate day in and day out. As a result, faithful Proactiv users are cheerfully applying benzoyl peroxide all over their faces once or twice a day, every day—one of the single most effective things you can do to keep *P. acnes* and inflammatory acne at bay.

USING BENZOYL PEROXIDE

Benzoyl peroxide is an intrinsically harsh chemical—an industrial bleach that has been used since the early part of the twentieth century to whiten flour and textiles. It can be very hard on the skin, causing redness, dryness, and scaling. It is also highly unstable and difficult to formulate; early dermatologic preparations had to be mixed just before they were used, then refrigerated or kept in special containers to maintain their effectiveness.

Arguably, one of the most significant recent developments in acne treatment has been the appearance of stable, effective, and cosmetically elegant over-the-counter benzoyl peroxide products, like Proactiv, that can be used consistently without ill effects. Even so, benzoyl peroxide retains a bad reputation among those who have used it improperly (i.e., sporadically, or solely as a spot treatment) and found it ineffective, or who have felt the unpleasant sting of its side effects and concluded they are allergic to it. But while a small percentage of people are indeed genuinely allergic to benzoyl peroxide, most of those who have had bad reactions have simply overused it. The trick—as with many of the most effective topical acne preparations—is to ease into it and use it consistently.

Benzoyl peroxide is available over the counter in creams, gels, lotions, and cleansers, in concentrations of 2.5 percent, 5 percent, and 10 percent. Begin with the lowest concentration, and apply it sparingly, once every other day, to the areas of skin where you have acne. If you have dark skin or sensitive skin, your best bet may be a benzoyl peroxide–containing wash or mask (for example, Neutrogena Clear Pore Cleanser/Mask) that you leave on your face for only a few minutes, then rinse off.

Your initial goal is to make sure you can use it once every day without experiencing any drying or other side effects. As your skin becomes accustomed to the benzoyl peroxide (doctors call this "hardening"), you can apply it twice a day. Be cautious about moving up to higher percentage products. The higher concentrations are much more likely to cause irritation, and they are only minimally more effective. According to a number of studies, benzoyl peroxide's antibacterial effects are similar at 2.5 percent, 5 percent, and 10 percent, and the *P. acnes* population remains low up to twenty-four hours after the product is applied. In other words, most users can do a good job of fighting acne by using the lowest concentration— and even if they use it only once a day.

If you do feel you need more firepower, you may want to try a 5 percent formula. But unless you have extremely oily skin (heavy sebum tends to dilute and "float off" any topical medicine), you should probably steer clear of higher percentages—

other than in a cleanser that you rinse off. The 10 percent, leave-on products are most appropriate for the very young and the extremely oily—say, teenage boys with really greasy skin.

If you experience any signs of true allergy—burning, blistering, crusting, itching, swelling, or severe redness—with any benzoyl peroxide product, stop using it immediately and consult a dermatologist. Because benzoyl peroxide is a bleaching agent, be careful to wash your hands after you apply it. If it rubs off on your clothes, your sheets, or your towels, it will leave a white patch; it may lighten your hair if it gets into the hairline.

SALICYLIC ACID

Salicylic acid is what is known as a kerolytic agent, which essentially means that it dissolves the protein in skin cells (keratinocytes). At very high concentrations, it is the standard ingredient in over-the-counter wart, callus, and corn removers. It appears in much lower percentages, from 0.5 percent to 2 percent, in acne products that exfoliate the surface of the skin and gradually work to loosen and expel comedones. Very gradually.

"The only things that really work for blackheads are prescription retinoids, like Retin-A," cautions O'Donoghue. "Salicylic acid will loosen comedones a little bit, but it's really just for someone with very mild acne."

"It's only mildly effective," agrees Dr. Albert Kligman, who estimates that a 2 percent salicylic acid acne product will take about three months to dislodge existing small comedones. And, he warns, "the big comedones won't come out at all." By comparison, he says, the prescription retinoid Tazorac (see page 71), can be expected to expel comedones—large or small—in about half the time, roughly six weeks.

But while salicylic acid products may have only a moderate effect on existing comedones, they can (if used consistently over the long term) help to keep sebaceous follicles clear of cellular buildup and prevent or minimize the creation of new comedones. Moreover, as surface exfoliants, they gently strip off the outermost layers of the skin's surface, improving its appearance and texture—and making it more receptive to any other acne-fighting medications you may be using. Finally, salicylic acid, which is chemically related to aspirin, is an anti-inflammatory agent that can help calm down the redness of pimples.

FINDING A GOOD SALICYLIC ACID PRODUCT.

You will frequently find salicylic acid referred to in advertising or on product labels as "beta hydroxy acid" (or BHA). Technically, this is a misnomer (chemists classify salicylic acid as an "aromatic compound"), but its use has become so common that the two terms are now virtually interchangeable.

Even though the vast majority of OTC acne medications contain salicylic acid, zeroing in on an effective, nonirritating one can be as tricky, if not more so, as finding a good benzoyl peroxide product. Because salicylic acid is not soluble in water, many of the products containing it are formulated with high concentrations of alcohol, which can be irritating to acne-prone skin. More crucially, salicylic acid is effective as an exfoliant only at concentrations of at least 1 percent, preferably 2 percent, and in an acid base, with a pH—a measure of acidity—between 3 and 4.

What it boils down to is this: For a salicylic acid product to have the greatest possible effect on your blemishes, it should contain 2 percent salicylic acid formulated at a pH of around 3 to 3.5.

The percentage is easy to determine; it will be stated on the label. It's not so simple to identify products with an appropriate pH. "I don't know how you're supposed to do *that*," says Shalita. "I guess it's sort of trial and error, and which ones your friends have used. The companies probably aren't going to tell you."

If you feel enterprising, you can actually investigate pH values for yourself, by using inexpensive paper testing strips that you dip into the product. The paper turns a color, which you match against a chart to determine the pH.

When I tried this myself, I found some of the results difficult to interpret. So I took a number of those products—cleansers, toners, and lotions—to my son's eighth-grade chemistry teacher, Erin Nieman, who subjected them to a far more accurate, computerized pH test. (Essentially, you dip a probe into a small sample and a digital pH reading pops up on the computer monitor.)

The results (shown on the charts on pages 208 and 211–212) were illuminating. Only some of the products fell into that optimum acid 3 to 3.5 pH range, thus measuring up in terms of being formulated for maximum possible exfoliating power. Many hovered at a pH of around 4—in other words, only minimally effective as an exfoliant. A few came up with readings of 6 or more.

It is probably only fair to mention that a number of these particular products were also loaded with various anti-inflammatory, antioxidant, or other possibly helpful (albeit unproven) ingredients, so they may, in fact, improve the condition of some people's acne. They're just not likely to be terribly effective exfoliants.

Alpha Hydroxy Acids

AHAs—alpha hydroxy acids—(the most common are glycolic and lactic acids) entered the consumer skin-care market in the early 1990s and are all but ubiquitous today, appearing in countless products promising to smooth, clear, and clean the skin. Like salicylic acid, alpha hydroxy acids work to loosen and strip dead cells from the surface of the skin, making it appear smoother and more even toned. AHAs are also humectants, which means that they draw moisture to the skin's surface.

AHAs are not oil soluble, so unlike salicylic acid, they do not penetrate as deeply into the oil-rich sebaceous follicle to exfoliate the cells that build up to create comedones. This means that they are not as likely to have as much of a direct impact on acne. But products containing AHAs (in particular glycolic acid) are often incorporated into commercial acne-fighting regimens, and many dermatologists feel that their surface exfoliating properties do work to improve breakouts.

In fact, medical peels, using high concentrations of glycolic acid, are frequently used by doctors as an office treatment for comedonal acne. By exfoliating superficial skin cells, a milder, over-the-counter glycolic acid lotion or toner can work as part of an overall acne treatment plan, preparing the skin for other acne products. Its moisturizing properties may also help counter some of the flaking caused by anti-acne ingredients such as benzoyl peroxide. And because it is water soluble, it is more likely than salicylic acid to be found in alcohol-free products.

"Glycolic acid probably does have a role in acne treatment, but there just haven't been any well-controlled studies," says Shalita. Plus, he adds, because AHAs are not regulated as acne drugs, "You never know exactly what you're getting. It varies from product to product, depending on how it's formulated, so nobody really knows what the heck is going on there."

RETINOL

The role of retinol, another ingredient frequently touted as an acne fighter, is equally murky. Retinol is the chemical name for vitamin A, the precursor (the mother chemical, if you will) of retinoic acid—which is the active ingredient in the prescription drug Retin-A (page 69), the gold standard in topical prescription acne treatment.

Retinol may be effective against acne because enzymes in the skin transform it into a chemical called retinaldehyde, which in turn transforms into trace amounts of retinoic acid. This means that, theoretically, retinol should have an effect that is similar to that of Retin-A, albeit milder. Whether it actually does is an open question. For starters, retinol is very unstable and difficult to package so that it maintains its effectiveness.

"The trick there is formulation," says Kligman. "If the concentration is high enough and it is stabilized, it should work. But what's available OTC—who knows? If it is made by a reputable drug house, and stabilized, and in sufficient concentration, it could have the same effect as retinoic acid. But there are hundreds of products out there with a dollop of retinol, and most of them don't work."

SULFUR AND RESORCINOL

Sulfur is one of the oldest of all drugs, and has been used as an acne treatment since antiquity. It is deadly to various strains of bacteria, as well as to fungi, parasites, and other microorganisms. And because it also softens and peels scaly skin, it has long been used to treat scaling inflammatory skin conditions such as seborrheic dermatitis and scabies.

Resorcinol, sulfur's sometime partner in acne medication, acts as a kerolytic agent (stripping off the outer surface of skin) and evidently boosts the effect of sulfur, although experts aren't sure exactly how the combination works. (Resorcinol alone is not effective in treating acne.) But resorcinol can be very irritating to some patients, and it may even discolor dark or black skin, so sensitive and dark-skinned patients are usually advised to avoid products containing it.

Many studies on acne patients have suggested that sulfur combined with benzoyl peroxide is more effective than either of the two alone, but since sulfur also increases sensitivity to benzoyl peroxide, drugs combining the ingredients must be used with care; some are available only by prescription.

In fact, acne experts differ on whether or not sulfur (with or without resorcinol or benzoyl peroxide) still belongs in the acne war chest. "Sulfur is out, out, *out!*" declares Plewig. "There is no place for it. It stinks and it's not effective, so why use it?"

"Sulfur is a *wonderful* ingredient," insists O'Donoghue. "It's a kerolytic, which means it takes off the horny layer; and it's antibacterial and anti-inflammatory. Sure, it's not as efficient against bacteria as benzoyl peroxide, and it's not as effective against comedones as the retinoids. But some people—like these blond, blue-eyed, ruddy folks—can't use benzoyl peroxide or Retin-A. Sulfur can be a good choice for them because it takes the inflammation out and does a nice job without overdrying. When I get the blond, ruddy people, I almost always grab one of the sulfur products."

Products containing sulfur are also good candidates as emergency spot treatments. Indeed, it's the key ingredient in a number of emergency acne treatments that have obtained something of a cult status, from the old drugstore favorite Acnomel, to pricey concoctions (Mario Badescu's Drying

Lotion and Sonya Dakar's Drying Potion), reputed to be the blemish-fighting secret weapons of supermodels and actresses.

"I know their mechanism is supposedly kerolytic and antibacterial, but I personally have seen such strong anti-inflammatory effects from sulfur and the sodium sulfacetamide products [page 85], that these are the main ones I recommend as spot treatments," says acne specialist Dr. Susan Bershad.

ACNE TREATMENT 101

Of course, no matter how effective any spot treatment may be, it is always a rear-guard action. The goal of acne treatment—whether it is a simple over-the-counter lotion, or the most potent of prescription drugs—is to keep pimples from forming in the first place. Treating the ones that have already emerged is largely futile. Yes, there are a few things you can do to keep them from getting worse (not picking is key) and a handful of things you can do to help them heal a little faster (see Chapter 11). But they're essentially lost causes. "Acne treatment is preventative, not something that you use to get rid of the pimples you've already got," emphasizes Shalita.

"Once you have a blemish, its really too late," agrees Bershad. "Acne treatments don't cure zits, and they are not meant to."

Consistency and persistence are the keys to acne prevention. Which means that even when your skin looks clear, you have to treat the parts that typically break out. Remember, as long as you have acne-prone skin, it is always producing excess sebum, it is always making those little time-bomb microcomedones, it is always hosting colonies of *P. acnes* bacteria. And it probably also has a hair-trigger inflammatory response.

Unfortunately, label instructions often mislead you. "The directions on a lot of these over-the-counter products say 'apply to affected area,' so people think the 'affected area' is just the spot where they actually have the pimple," points out Shalita. "But it's the whole area of skin."

A light hand is also critical. "Most people want to get rid of their acne yesterday," notes O'Donoghue. "So they go out and buy Oxy 10, and cleansing grains to wash with, and maybe an astringent with alcohol, and before you know it, their faces are like raw meat."

Gentle cleansing is particularly important.

"Aggressive cleansing in general is one of the biggest mistakes people make," says Bershad. "It doesn't improve your acne, and it's detrimental in a lot of ways. In the first place, irritating the skin reduces tolerance to effective acne medication. If you start with an irritated surface, acne medicines are going to cause another burden of skin irritation. Also, overly aggressive cleansing causes skin swelling. And when you have skin swelling, it tightens the pores, trapping stuff in the lower portion of the follicle. And that can make the acne even worse."

Bershad advises women to steer clear of products marketed directly to teens, whose complexions tend to be much oilier and thus less vulnerable to the relatively high concentrations of alcohol that are typically found in teen acne medications. "A lot of these products geared to teens are too drying for older skin. Women use them, and their skin gets irritated, and then they go and use moisturizers that are really heavy, and that makes their acne worse."

Both Bershad and O'Donoghue also advise against mechanical exfoliants such as loofahs or ground-up nuts or minerals, all of which can abrade facial skin—and may even cause additional damage. "Boy, years ago, when I started practicing, we used to use these really abrasive cleansers—like apricot scrubs," recalls O'Donoghue. "They were a great gimmick. But then all these patients started coming in with calcium deposits below the surface of the skin. The particles got into the pores, and the skin reacted just like an oyster making a pearl!"

AN ACNE REGIMEN

There is no one right way to put together an over-the-counter acne treatment regimen. "One of the main principles of acne treatment is that each person reacts differently to various agents and different products. And patients have different preferences," says Bershad. "What works well for one woman won't necessarily work for the next one. It all depends."

The simplest, bare-bones advice is to find a benzoyl peroxide product that you like and a salicylic acid product that you like and build them into a cleansing and treatment regimen that suits you—making sure to use the benzoyl peroxide and the salicylic acid once or twice a day, each.

Bershad further suggests using benzoyl peroxide and salicylic acid products at different times of the day, for example, one at bedtime and one in the morning. "Or at least wait ten to twenty minutes between if you're using one on top of the other. The reason is that benzoyl peroxide has the effect of oxidizing other compounds, and acid formulations, like retinoic acid, are vulnerable to that. And although I don't think it's been studied, it's possible that salicylic acid could also be inactivated by benzoyl peroxide."

The greatest range of choice for either product will be found among acne-fighting cleansers. The majority of these contain salicylic acid, and, in fact, one of the easiest possible acne regimens is to wash with a salicylic acid cleanser and follow with a leave-on benzoyl peroxide product.

But to get the most out of any anti-acne soap or cleanser, whether it incorporates benzoyl peroxide or salicylic acid, you

have to keep it on your face long enough for the active ingredients to get into the skin. How long is that? Good question.
"You know, the studies just haven't been done," says Bershad.

"What most people do with cleansers is just rinse them off
right away," says Shalita. "We say lather up and keep it on for a
couple of minutes. Salicylic acid is lipid soluble, and it penetrates
fairly quickly, so if you leave it on a few minutes it does the trick."

But who actually has the patience to keep a cleanser on her
face for "a couple of minutes"? And even if you do, medicated
cleansers may still pose other problems. "If you are using a
benzoyl peroxide or salicylic acid soap all over your face, that
area under the eye where the skin is so thin and tender can get
really sore and irritated," cautions O'Donoghue, who generally
advises acne patients to skip the acne cleansers and instead
wash with gentle detergents. "I would rather see a patient use
Dove on her whole face and then put the acne medicines just
where she needs them. Also, while it may be okay to use an
acne soap with an over-the-counter acne lotion, if you are
using an acne soap with a prescription acne treatment, you
can end up being chapped and unable to use the prescription
lotion where you need it."

WHEN TO TURN TO A DERMATOLOGIST

Despite the fact that many women with acne can get good results with over-the counter remedies, it is probably always best
for any adult who has acne to see a dermatologist at least initially, if for no other reason than to get a baseline diagnosis.
There is always the possibility that what you have is not true
acne, but one of the acne-like disorders. And frankly, the older
you get, the likelier you are to acquire peculiar little epidermal
eruptions—including certain skin cancers—that can look for all

the world like acne pimples. Or your breakouts may be a symptom of some other, underlying medical condition. In either case, the sooner a doctor figures out what is going on and starts you on appropriate treatment, the better off you will be.

You should always head straight to a dermatologist if your acne is severe—particularly if it is leaving scars or other lingering marks, such as the pigmented spots that commonly appear on dark skin. In those cases, the prescription medicines only a physician can supply will work faster and more effectively than anything you can get over the counter.

Similarly, if you have anything else going on with your skin in addition to acne (rosacea, psoriasis, perioral dermatitis, rashes of any sort, pigmentation irregularities, or extensive sun damage, to name just a few of the possibilities), your best bet is a dermatologist; treating two conditions simultaneously can be very tricky.

Another sign that you need medical help (in fact, this is a serious red flag, not to be ignored at any cost) is if you have acne in an unusual location, such as your scalp, your armpits, or your groin. There are some rare, but very serious, forms of acne that sometimes show up in odd places on your body; they absolutely require a doctor's care. And the sooner the better. Some of these conditions can get so out of hand that they require surgery and skin grafts to correct.

All that being said, if you do turn first to over-the-counter medication for your acne, you should start to see results of some kind in six to eight weeks—if not actual clearing, at least a significant reduction in the size and number of inflammatory lesions. (Comedones typically take longer; it can take up to three months or more for OTC remedies to make much of a dent in existing blackheads or whiteheads.) If you are truly being consistent and nothing has happened by eight or ten weeks, and especially if you are getting new lesions, please make an appointment with a dermatologist.

Chapter Six

——◁◇▷——

Prescription Treatment

THE ARRAY OF PRESCRIPTION DRUGS now available for treating acne is nothing short of remarkable. There are dozens of different medicines, and hundreds of conceivable ways they can be combined into individually tailored regimens.

"There is a place for all of them," says Dr. Susan Bershad. "Those of us who specialize in acne can use every single product that's out there."

Even for very severe acne, most dermatologists do not immediately turn to Accutane (Chapter 7), the only drug that simultaneously battles all of the major factors contributing to acne: comedones, bacteria, inflammation, and oil production. Similarly, they do not routinely jump right in with drugs such as birth control pills or anti-androgens that address the hormonal causes of acne (Chapter 8)—although doctors today are increasingly likely to question women acne patients about potential hormonal influences when they take an initial medical history, and they will investigate further if it appears warranted.

Typically, they start out by turning first to the two mainstays in acne treatment: topical retinoids, a group of medicines that work to expel comedones and prevent new ones from forming, and antibiotics, either taken orally or applied directly to the face, to fight bacteria and inflammation.

TOPICAL RETINOIDS

Topical retinoids are the foundation treatment for most common forms of acne. A large class of drugs derived from vitamin A (retinol is the chemical name for vitamin A), retinoids are used to treat many different skin disorders and are widely regarded as among the most important of all dermatologic drugs. They have been a pillar of acne therapy since 1971, when the original formulation, Retin-A, was introduced.

It would be hard to exaggerate the importance that acne experts attach to topical retinoids. Leading researchers such as Albert Kligman (sometimes called the Father of Retin-A), SUNY's Alan Shalita, and the University of Pennsylvania's James Leyden, all with decades of experience in treating acne, are practically evangelical on the subject. They say flatly that virtually anyone with acne or acne-prone skin can benefit from topical retinoids.

And yet many doctors, including many dermatologists, rarely prescribe topical retinoids for their acne patients. Some simply wimp out, says Kligman, because they are unwilling to take the time and attention needed to nurse patients through the tricky early weeks of therapy when side effects such as red, peeling skin are common. "They don't want to get called off the golf course," he scoffs.

According to Shalita, many other doctors prescribe retinoids only for non-inflammatory acne (blackheads and whiteheads), in the mistaken belief that they are ineffective against inflamed papules and pustules—or that they will, in fact, only make inflamed lesions worse by aggravating the inflammation. "One of the great myths for many years in dermatology has been that retinoids are only for comedones, and that you need something else for inflammatory acne," he explains. "Well, Jim Leyden and I have been lecturing for twenty-five years on the effects of retinoids on inflammatory acne. And over the years there have been numerous good clinical trials showing really impressive reductions in inflammatory lesions using just retinoids alone—without any other agents. Now, we think a retinoid should be used in conjunction with an antibacterial agent; you get the best results that way. But the bottom line is that retinoids work, and work well, on inflammatory acne."

Retinoids are effective against both forms of acne, he explains, because by keeping the sebaceous follicles free of comedones, they strike acne at the very outset, at the magic "precursor" stage. "The key to acne is in the follicles. To get acne, a follicle has to respond to the stimulus of the precursor lesion, the microcomedo. If the cells lining the follicle wall no longer plug up to create microcomedones, then you don't have acne."

Retinoids do not achieve these results by peeling the skin. Despite a common misconception, they are not exfoliants, like alpha hydroxy or salicylic acids, which gradually strip off the top layers of skin. Retinoids are instead what might be called skin cell "normalizers," hormone-like chemical messengers whose molecules bind to receptors in the nucleus of each skin cell to change the way those cells behave. In acne-prone skin, retinoids essentially turn abnormal keratinocytes that accumulate and stick together in follicles, into normal keratinocytes that exit the follicles in a normal fashion. In similar fashion, they help to "normalize" aging, sun-damaged skin cells, which is why they are also used to treat superficial signs of aging such as fine wrinkles and blotchy age spots. In both cases, irritation and excessive peeling are side effects, not part of the therapeutic process.

Unfortunately, the more potent the retinoid is, the more

likely it is to produce side effects. The original form of Retin-A was a powerful solution that wowed researchers by causing comedones to practically pop out of patients' skin before their very eyes. But the blistering potion—"like liquid fire," says Shalita—left patients' faces raw. Newer versions have been formulated with an eye toward balancing speed and effectiveness against irritation. As a general rule, those that are less irritating tend to work a little less quickly and effectively. Nonetheless, they all attack acne in essentially the same manner—by altering the environment in the sebaceous follicle so that cells no longer clump together. According to experts (and a number of clinical trials directly comparing different versions), they all produce about the same results over the long run. "It doesn't matter so much which one you use. They all do the job," says Shalita. "The important thing, if you have acne, is to be on a retinoid, period."

RETINOID OPTIONS

The choices among topical retinoids available in the United States today include several variations of the original Retin-A, and two so-called "synthetic retinoids," which are not derived from retinol, but which act on similar receptors in skin cells and thus behave like retinoids. (Other retinoids, including a topical version of Accutane, can be found in other countries but have not been approved by the Food and Drug Administration for use in the United States.)

Tretinoin (Retin-A, Renova, Avita)
Tretinoin (or retinoic acid) is the generic name for Retin-A, the first retinoid used on acne and still regarded by dermatologists as the gold standard in topical acne treatment. As well as

treating acne, tretinoin also improves the appearance of aged skin by correcting irregular pigmentation and smoothing the fine lines that are signs of sun damage to collagen in the dermis—the middle layer of the skin. Renova, an emollient-based version of Retin-A, was the first topical drug ever approved by the Food and Drug Administration to reverse visible signs of aging.

Retin-A is available in several different strengths and in a cream, gel, or solution base. An alternate form, called Retin-A Micro, packages the active ingredient (tretinoin) in tiny "microsponges" that release the chemical into the skin gradually, with less irritation. Yet another version of tretinoin, called Avita, chemically bundles the active ingredient into minicapsules that act similarly, releasing the drug slowly into the skin.

Because exposure to sunlight degrades tretinoin, many dermatologists recommend that you apply it only at night. But if, for some reason, you want to use it in the daytime, you can—with care. "The problems with the sun have been grossly exaggerated," says Shalita. "Yes, it's true that vitamin A acid is unstable when exposed to ultraviolet light. But, the way most people use it, by the time you put it on, have breakfast, and do whatever else you're going to do in the morning, it's already been absorbed into the skin. You'd have to be really sunbathing for the light to affect it. Plus, tretinoin in microsponges [Retin-A Micro, Avita] is more stable because it's encapsulated and the sun won't affect it."

Tretinoin is also inactivated by benzoyl peroxide, so if you are using a benzoyl peroxide product and tretinoin together as part of a combination regimen, doctors usually advise applying them at different times of day—say, one in the morning and the other at night.

Adapalene *(Differin)*

The synthetic retinoid adapalene, introduced in the United States in 1996 under the trade name Differin, is generally regarded as the least irritating as well as the most cosmetically elegant of the topical retinoids; it also has anti-inflammatory properties. It has become extremely popular with women patients, in part because it can easily be worn under makeup. Unlike tretinoin, it is not affected by either sunlight or benzoyl peroxide, making it far more convenient to use. It is available in cream, gel, and solution form, and in pledgets—individually packaged towelettes impregnated with the solution. Unlike tretinoin and tazarotene (discussed below), adapalene has not been proven to be effective for treating sun-damaged skin. Nonetheless, some dermatologists feel that if used consistently, over time it should have similar skin-smoothing effects.

Tazarotene *(Tazorac, Avage)*

Tazarotene (trade name Tazorac) is another synthetic retinoid; it was approved by the FDA in 1997 for treating psoriasis, and shortly thereafter for acne. In 2002, the FDA approved a 0.1 percent tazarotene cream called Avage for use, like Renova, as a treatment for signs of photo-aging.

Tazarotene is generally regarded as the fastest-working, yet most potentially irritating, of the topical retinoids. According to Allergan, the company that makes it, tests comparing Tazorac to Differin have demonstrated that Tazorac reduces comedonal acne by 34 percent in the first four weeks of use and by 68 percent by the end of week twelve, while Differin produces a 7 percent reduction at week four, and a 36 percent reduction at week twelve. Also, says Bershad, "In my experience, tazarotene is the only topical drug that visibly shrinks pores." (Theoretically, all topical retinoids should gradually

reduce pore size as they normalize follicles and stimulate collagen production in the surrounding tissues; but generally, the
effects are so subtle that you can't tell.)

USING TOPICAL RETINOIDS

The key to using retinoids safely is to start slow and low. "If
you are a first-time Retin-A patient, and you put it on every
night, you are going to be in *tears*," warns dermatologist Laurie
Polis. "There are very few people who can start out handling a
retinoid every night."

- Start with a low percentage (for example 0.025 percent
  Retin-A, or Differin cream) and apply it sparingly every
  other night, or every third night. If your skin seems irritated, slow down even more—applying it only every
  fourth of fifth night. It typically takes somewhere
  between three to six weeks for the skin to become sufficiently resilient to allow more frequent use. But it can
  take even longer, especially if you are applying it only a
  few times a week. "You have to effect an anatomic
  change in the skin," says Polis. "That can take six
  weeks—or six months. You have to be really patient."

- Use a gentle cleanser, such as Cetaphil liquid, to wash
  your face. Then dry carefully and wait ten or fifteen
  minutes before applying the retinoid. If your face is
  moist, the medicine will penetrate too quickly, increasing the potential for irritation. Apply sparingly. The
  classic guideline is to squeeze a pea-sized dot onto the
  tip of one finger, lightly dab small amounts on the forehead, cheeks, and chin; then smooth it all over.

- For the first few weeks, at least, avoid all other potentially irritating topical medicines, such as benzoyl peroxide, salicylic acids, toners, and topical antibiotics; these can be added to your routine, if needed, after your skin becomes accustomed to the retinoid.

- Use a moisturizer to combat irritation or peeling. "I definitely recommend moisturizers for patients on retinoids," says Bershad. "Finding an appropriate one is usually a matter of trial and error. Patients usually start with an oil-free moisturizer that's specific for acne-prone skin. Then, if that doesn't seem emollient enough, they can try any non-comedogenic facial lotion, preferably fragrance-free. I usually have them apply the moisturizer first, then the topical retinoid. Or they can put them on at different times of day. But I would not apply a moisturizer after the retinoid, because then you may actually be occluding the medication, making it stronger. Wait for the moisturizer to vanish before putting on the retinoid so that you're not applying the retinoid to a wet surface."

- At two to three weeks, your acne may look worse. This is what doctors call a "flare," an inflammatory blowup of invisible micro-comedones. This is actually a positive sign—that those invisible comedones are being expelled—so don't give up.

- Apply a broad-spectrum, minimum SPF 15, sunscreen every morning on treated skin, even if you don't expect to go outside, and even if you have naturally dark skin and don't customarily use sun protection. Retinoids are not photosensitizing in the true sense of the word (a photosensitizing agent is one that, when applied to the skin, absorbs sunlight in such a way that it chemically damages skin cells). But, retinoids do thin the outer layers of the skin, making you more vulnerable to ultraviolet rays, and thus increasing the chances that you will burn.

- Be patient. The amount of time that it takes to see results varies from person to person, but it can take as long as three to four months of consistent use to see obvious improvement in your acne. Unfortunately, because progress is so gradual, and side effects are so common, many people give up on retinoids long before they see any benefits.

- If you are pregnant or considering becoming pregnant, talk to your doctor about whether you can continue to use a topical retinoid. The patient package information for all topical retinoids warns against their use during pregnancy because all known *oral* retinoids (such as Accutane, or high doses of vitamin A) can cause birth defects. Although topical retinoids have not been shown to affect developing fetuses, most doctors strongly advise pregnant or breast-feeding women to avoid them. Says Bershad, "I don't think any dermatologist should prescribe topical retinoids to a pregnant or lactating woman."

RETINOIDS AND DARK SKIN

Many dermatologists are especially cautious about using topical retinoids on dark-skinned patients, because they fear that retinoid-induced irritation may increase the tendency of dark skin to develop the lingering spots of post-inflammatory hyperpigmentation. Indeed, dermatologists who treat dark-skinned patients are leery of *any* anti-acne medicine they feel may irritate the skin. However, those who are experienced in using retinoids maintain that not only can they be safely employed on dark skin, but that, used correctly, they actually counteract hyperpigmentation.

As always with any potentially irritating ingredient, the key is to take it slowly, following the same careful guidelines (discussed above) as all retinoid patients. Dr. Susan Taylor, of New York's Skin of Color Institute, also cautions that it is particularly important for doctors who are prescribing retinoids for dark-skinned patients to simultaneously treat any existing inflammation.

"The first thing I do is look for inflammation, and if there are a lot of inflamed papules and nodules, I will go immediately to an oral antibiotic to get that under control. I also inquire very carefully about dryness or oiliness, and about the other products the patient is using, to make sure she stops using anything else that might be irritating—like benzoyl peroxide, or glycolic or salicylic acid, or strong cleansers. Then I start with a low-strength retinoid. I find that Differin or Differin cream is the least drying. In fact, the cream is a little moisturizing, which is wonderful."

According to one small study of fourteen dark-skinned acne patients (ten African American, four Hispanic), even Tazorac, which is generally regarded as the most irritating of the topical retinoids, can be uneventfully used on dark skin if carefully introduced. Each night, study subjects washed their faces with gentle Cetaphil liquid cleanser. Ten to twenty minutes later, they mixed a pea-sized dot of 0.05 percent tazarotene gel with a similar pea-sized portion of Cetaphil moisturizer and applied the mixture to their faces. They washed with Cetaphil again in the morning and applied sunscreen. They used no antibiotics and applied nothing else to their skin beyond the cleanser, the retinoid with the moisturizer, and the sunscreen.

By the end of two weeks, five patients stopped using the moisturizer altogether and switched to the undiluted gel (the rest stayed with the mix). At the end of eight weeks, all of them showed dramatic reductions in inflammation and number of acne lesions; none complained of irritation or burning.

ORAL ANTIBIOTICS

Widely used to treat acne since the 1950s, broad-spectrum oral antibiotics have been the traditional workhorse weapons against inflammatory acne ever since. They operate in two ways: preemptively, by destroying inflammation-provoking *P. acnes* bacteria; and directly, by curbing inflammatory chemicals produced by the body, thus taming existing inflammation. These are such important aspects of acne treatment that some patients spend literally years taking antibiotics, faithfully downing daily "maintenance" doses to keep inflammation at a low burn and their breakouts under control.

But increasingly, acne experts are questioning that strategy. Antibiotics become progressively less effective the longer they are used. Like children repeatedly treated with antibiotics for chronic ear infections, acne patients become resistant to their drugs because *P. acnes* and other bacteria in the body mutate into resistant strains that no longer respond to the medicine. And that tendency appears to be sharply on the upswing. According to one review of the medical literature, over the eighteen-year period between 1978 and 1996, the reported rate of *P. acnes* resistance to antibiotics more than tripled, from 20 percent to 62 percent of acne patients developing resistant bacteria from their treatment.

Accordingly, many dermatologists today sharply limit antibiotic therapy to a relatively short period (no more than six months, says Shalita; as little as ten to fifteen days for some patients, suggests Bershad). The goal is to quickly get acute inflammation under control. The antibiotic is typically prescribed in conjunction with a topical retinoid, which is then continued over the long term, as maintenance therapy to keep new comedones from forming. If needed, another antimicrobial agent, such as benzoyl peroxide, is brought in to keep *P. acnes* and inflammation under control over the long term. (Because bacteria do not become resistant to benzoyl peroxide, it can be used indefinitely.)

Any antibiotic will kill *P. acnes* in a test tube, but only a handful are capable of penetrating the oil-rich sebaceous follicles to reach the acne-aggravating *P. acnes* that dwell and multiply there. (Penicillin, for example, is not used to treat acne because it does not get into the follicles.) The oral antibiotics prescribed for acne generally come from one of two families, the tetracyclines (including the so-called "second-generation" tetracyclines) and the macrolides.

Tetracycline *(Sumycin, Achromycin V, others)*

Tetracyline is the oral antibiotic most frequently prescribed for acne. It is popular with doctors and patients alike, because it is both inexpensive and effective. But it can be an irksome drug to use, with a long list of stipulations and drawbacks.

Because tetracycline has a very short half-life (that means it dissipates quickly inside the body), you must take it several times a day in order to maintain a constant therapeutic level in your bloodstream. Food and milk interfere with its absorption, so you have to take it on an empty stomach—thirty to sixty minutes before a meal or two hours afterward. It also cannot be taken with calcium or iron supplements, or with antacids containing magnesium, aluminum, or iron; all of these minerals render it ineffective.

Tetracycline boosts the effects of some drugs, notably lithium and anticoagulants, so you need to talk to your doctor about adjusting the doses of other medicines while you're taking it. Also, remember that lithium and some other drugs are acne promoters (see Chapter 4); they can cancel out the acne-fighting activity of tetracycline—as well as other acne drugs.

Tetracycline has a number of potential side effects. By destroying normal, beneficial flora in the body, it may leave you vulnerable to opportunistic organisms such as those that cause vaginal yeast infections—which are common in women taking tetracycline. Its effects on the normal bacterial environment in the stomach may also interfere with the manner in which the hormones in oral contraceptives are absorbed. Hypothetically, this could lead to contraceptive failure, particularly during the first four or five weeks of tetracycline therapy while the body adjusts to the drug. That is why doctors and pharmacists frequently advise women who use the Pill to switch to an alternate form of birth control while taking tetracycline.

Tetracycline is also phototoxic, which means that once it is in the skin, it will absorb energy from sunlight, causing damage to skin cells. You need to be scrupulous about sun protection when taking it.

Do not take tetracycline if you are pregnant or breast-feeding, and do not give it to children under thirteen years old; the drug is deposited in the developing skeletons of fetuses and young children, causing tooth discoloration and hampering bone growth. Occasionally, tetracycline can cause other serious side effects, including headache, blurred vision, and a lupus-like syndrome. (Patients who have lupus or a family history of lupus should not use tetracycline.)

Doxycycline (Adoxa, Doryx, Monodox, Vibramycin)

Doxycycline and minocycline (discussed below) are the two second-generation tetracyclines most frequently prescribed for acne. Both are more expensive than the original form, and they have similar side effects. However, second-generation tetracyclines are much more convenient to use. They have longer half-lives, which means they do not need to be taken as frequently, and they can be taken with food. In fact, some doctors recommend that patients do take doxycycline and minocycline with meals to reduce the chances of their causing digestive upset or esophageal inflammation.

Recently, doctors have investigated a promising alternate form of doxycyline, called Periostat, for acne. Periostat is an anti-inflammatory drug that has been used for more than twenty years by dentists to combat periodontal gum disease, which, like acne, is an inflammatory condition. It is typically prescribed in very low doses, thus producing far fewer side effects than other forms of doxycycline. In a 2002 study conducted by the dermatology departments of the University of Florida and the University of West Virginia, patients with moderate acne who received 20 milligrams of periostat twice a day for six months (much less than the typical 100 to 200 milligram daily doxycycline dose for acne), saw significant improvement in both their inflammatory acne and (surprisingly) also in their numbers of comedones.

Minocycline (Dynacin, Minocin)

Minocycline is considered by many dermatologists to be the most potent of the common anti-acne oral antibiotics. It penetrates sebaceous glands extremely well, and appears to work more rapidly on bacteria and inflammation than either tetracycline or doxycycline. Its other advantage is that of all the oral antibiotics used for acne, it appears thus far to have the lowest potential for developing antibiotic resistance.

In general, minocycline is considered safe. However, over the long term it can have serious side effects. In some instances, patients who have been on minocycline therapy for many months and have accumulated a high total dose in their bodies have developed spots of a blue-gray pigment in areas where their skin has been inflamed (including the sites of old acne lesions) or exposed to the sun.

Erythromycin (Eryc, Ery-Tab, others)

Erythromycin, one of what are known as the macrolide antibiotics, is the most common alternative to the tetracyclines in treating acne. It is considered less effective against inflammation, and regarded as more likely to produce resistant strains of *P. acnes*. But it can be used in situations when tetracycline would be harmful, such as during pregnancy and while breast-feeding. It can be taken with or without food.

TOPICAL ANTIBIOTICS

Like antibiotics taken by mouth, topical antibiotics that are applied directly to the skin both attack *P. acnes* and quell existing inflammation. They offer one distinct advantage over systemic antibiotics in that they do not affect the whole body, so they do not present the same risk of side effects. However, they are generally less effective than oral antibiotics in reducing inflamed lesions, and they are considered more likely to promote bacterial resistance. The two most common topical antibiotics prescribed for acne are clindamycin and erythromycin; topical tetracycline has not proven itself effective against acne.

Clindamycin *(Cleocin T, Clindagel, Clinda-Derm, ClindaMax)*
Clindamycin is the most frequently used of the two; it is available in a number of forms. For example, Cleocin T, one of the more popular brands, comes in three forms: a mild lotion for patients with dry skin, a gel that can be used under cosmetics, and pledgets (individually packaged towelettes impregnated with the solution). Galderma, the same company that makes the mild cleanser Cetaphil and the "kinder, gentler" retinoid Differin, produces a version called Clindagel, which is an oil- and alcohol-free gel that spreads easily, absorbs rapidly without leaving a residue, and can be used under makeup.

Erythromycin *(A/T/S, Akne-Mycin, Dermamycin, Emgel, Ery-Sol, Erycette, Eryderm, Erygel, Erymax, Staticin, T-Stat)*
Topical erythromycin is less expensive than clindamycin, and it is available in a number of different formulations. However, like oral erythromycin, it is among the antibiotics regarded as more likely to promote bacterial resistance. Two popular forms are Emgel, a gel that goes on smoothly and is invisible under makeup; and Akne-Mycin, an ointment in a creamy, moisturizing base that the manufacturer claims is particularly good for acne patients who are also using other topical agents such as tretinoin or benzoyl peroxide, or for those who have eczema or who live in cold climates.

PRESCRIPTION BENZOYL PEROXIDE

Topical benzoyl peroxide, the *P. acnes*–fighting champ of non-prescription acne treatment (pages 51-55), is also a major combatant in the prescription acne wars—and for the same excellent reasons: Benzoyl peroxide ruthlessly suppresses *P. acnes*, without ever losing its effectiveness because bacteria cannot become resistant to it. And it has a mild comedolytic effect, which means that it can also help in the battle against comedones.

Benzoyl peroxide is frequently used in combination with topical retinoids (the peerless comedo terminators), as either an alternative or an adjunct to antibiotics (the bacteria and inflammation busters). However, because of benzoyl peroxide's tendency to irritate the skin, doctors typically wait four to six weeks (or longer, if necessary) before incorporating benzoyl peroxide into a regimen that also includes a retinoid. Dermatologists also generally advise against using the two agents at the same time of day—particularly if you are using topical tretinoin (such as Retin-A, Retin-A Micro, or Avita), because benzoyl peroxide inactivates tretinoin. However, even if you are using one of the synthetic retinoids (adapalene or tazarotene, which are not affected by benzoyl peroxide), it is generally still a good idea to apply them at different times; if you use more than one of these strong topical agents together, they have a tendency to dilute one another, potentially making each less effective individually. "I tell patients to do everything in the bathroom, then wait and put on the retinoid right before you go to sleep," says Marianne O'Donoghue.

Benzoyl Peroxide Lotions, Gels, Creams, and Washes
(Brevoxyl, Triaz, Clinac BPO)

Prescription benzoyl peroxide medicines are similar to over-the-counter formulas in that they are available in a variety of strengths (from 3 to 10 percent) and in different vehicles, including cleansers, which doctors may prescribe for patients with sensitive skin who can't tolerate a leave-on benzoyl peroxide medicine. The Triaz brand gels, lotions, and cleansers all also contain zinc, which, it is believed, may enhance the inflammation-fighting properties of benzoyl peroxide. Clinac BPO is a gel that also includes a topical oil-dispersing agent, which means that it can help you look less greasy—although it will not affect the amount of sebum produced by your sebaceous glands.

Benzoyl Peroxide–Antibiotic Combinations (Benzamycin, BenzaClin, Duac)

Among the most effective of all medicines for inflammatory acne are topical drugs that contain both benzoyl peroxide and an antibiotic in a single product. These combination drugs are awesome acne fighters; a number of studies have shown that they are far better at reducing existing lesions and preventing new ones from forming than either benzoyl peroxide or an antibiotic alone. Because they work through different mechanisms, together they deliver a powerful double punch to bacteria and inflammation. Yet, at the same time, because each agent is typically present at a somewhat lower concentration than it would be when used alone, together they are less likely to produce irritation or other unwelcome side effects. (In fact, it appears that the antibiotic may actually help suppress any redness or irritation caused by the benzoyl peroxide.) Perhaps most critically of all, benzoyl peroxide kills bacteria so quickly that they do not have the opportunity to produce antibiotic-resistant strains; emerging mutants are killed off before they can multiply and establish themselves.

OTHER PRESCRIPTION CHOICES

While retinoids, antibiotics, and benzoyl peroxide are the chief weapons in the acne war chest (with Accutane and hormonal treatment constituting the specialized heavy armament), a number of other prescription drugs and treatments offer additional means of tweaking therapy for individual circumstances.

Azelaic Acid *(Azelex, Finacea, Finevin)*

Azelaic acid is a naturally occurring substance (found in cereal grains), with antibacterial effects that can slow the growth of *P. acnes* and reduce inflammation in mild or moderate acne. It is also a bleaching agent that inhibits the production of the skin pigment melanin, making it particularly helpful in counteracting post-inflammatory hyperpigmentation.

Azelaic acid does not suppress *P. acnes* bacteria as quickly or as thoroughly as either benzoyl peroxide or antibiotics, but it is relatively gentle on the skin. It produces far less dryness and scaling than benzoyl peroxide, making it an attractive option for patients with sensitive skin, with rosacea, or who are allergic to benzoyl peroxide. And bacteria do not become resistant to azelaic acid, so it can be used as an alternative to antibiotics for long-term therapy. Azelaic acid is available in the United States in topical creams and gels under the trade names Azelex, Finacea, and Finevin.

Sodium Sulfacetimide (Klaron, Plexion, Rosac, Rosanil, Sulfacet, Novacet, Clenia, Rosex, Rosula)

Sodium sulfacetimide belongs to a class of drugs known as sulfonamides, which inhibit the growth of bacteria by interfering with certain enzymes that the microbes need in order to grow and multiply. It is a highly soluble agent that can be easily formulated into nonirritating, alcohol-free lotions; it is often used in drugs to treat eye infections. Topical skin preparations containing sodium sulfacetimide are prescribed both for acne and rosacea. These can be particularly helpful for acne patients who are easily irritated by other topical medications, or who are natural "flushers and blushers," showing early signs of rosacea.

Klaron is a 10 percent sodium sulfacetimide lotion; Plexion, Sulfacet, Clenia, Rosac, and Novacet all contain sodium sulfacetimide in combination with sulfur, which through its anti-inflammatory and anti-kerolytic effects is thought to boost the effects of the sodium sulfacetimide and help reduce comedones, papules, and pustules. Rosac adds sunscreen to the mix to protect skin from ultraviolet light. Another acne and rosacea preparation called Rosula includes moisturizing urea to further soothe red or irritated skin.

Metronidazole (MetroGel, MetroLotion, MetroCream, Noritate)

Metronidazole is an anti-infective agent that kills organisms by interacting with their DNA to destroy cell nuclei. In its oral form (Flagyl is one of the more familiar trade names), metronidazole is used to fight urinary, genital, and digestive tract infections. Several topical forms (MetroGel, MetroLotion, MetroCream, and Noritate) are used to control rosacea by reducing redness and inflammatory papules and pustules. The FDA has not approved these medicines for *acne vulgaris*, but sometimes doctors prescribe them as a gentle weapon against inflamed acne lesions.

Nicotinamide *(Nicomide)*

Nicotinamide is a form of niacin, part of the vitamin B complex. (Niacin deficiency causes pellagra, a nutritional disorder that affects skin by causing itching and inflammation.) Applied topically, it has anti-inflammatory activity and may also reduce the proliferation of skin cells in the follicle—two effects that make it potentially useful against acne. A prescription tablet called Nicomide, containing nicotinamide, zinc, and folic acid, has been approved by the FDA for treating acne. A few researchers have also investigated the effect of topical nicotinamide on acne; in one trial, it proved to have the same impact on inflammatory lesions as the topical antibiotic clindamycin.

Sulfones *(Dapsone)*

The sulfones are a group of powerful drugs used on a variety of severe skin conditions. One of the sulfones, Dapsone, is a leprosy treatment that has both anti-inflammatory effects and antimicrobial activity against *P. acnes*. Although it is not FDA approved for treating acne, some dermatologists occasionally prescribe oral Dapsone for patients with extremely severe cystic breakouts, who, for one reason or another, cannot tolerate more conventional acne treatments. Researchers have also investigated a topical Dapsone gel for use on acne. Warning: Dapsone is highly toxic and can produce serious side effects. Patients taking it require careful monitoring of their liver and kidney function, with frequent blood and urine tests.

LIGHT THERAPY

In 2002, the Food and Drug Administration approved two new acne treatments that exploit the therapeutic powers of light to battle breakouts. While both are still in their infancy and are undergoing a succession of further tests, each appears to offer a promising new avenue to clear skin.

Blue Light Treatment (ClearLight)

The proprietary ClearLight system (made by a company called Lumenis) is a lamp that emits a beam of blue light at 410 to 420 nanometers, a wavelength that activates certain pigments in *P. acnes* bacteria. These pigments, called porphyrins, absorb the light, producing a chemical reaction that kills the bacteria. Unlike damaging ultraviolet light, the blue light does not burn the skin or increase the risk of skin cancer.

"This is a light similar to what we use to treat jaundice in newborns," explains Dr. Alan Shalita, who was one of the chief investigators in the clinical trials leading to FDA approval of the device. "It's a very high intensity light that doesn't have any side effects that we can see. And it does appear to destroy the bacteria in the skin."

ClearLight is a possible alternative to antibiotics—a drug-free means of treating moderate inflammatory acne. It does not work on severe cystic eruptions, and it doesn't seem to have an effect on very mild or noninflamed breakouts. (Evidently, there has to be a certain amount of bacteria present in the skin to produce the necessary amount of porphyrins to absorb the light.)

A typical course of ClearLight treatment consists of a month of fifteen-minute sessions, twice a week. According to the results of the initial trials, patients whose acne responded to the light saw anywhere from a 50 to 70 percent reduction in the number of acne lesions after a month. Their acne continued to improve for another month afterward, with some experiencing even more clearing over the following three months.

"I don't think this is a cure for acne," comments Shalita. "But it is a noninvasive, nonchemical treatment, so that maybe, if you used it with Retin-A, you wouldn't have to use antibiotics."

Laser Treatment (Smoothbeam)

The Smoothbeam laser approved for acne treatment is what is known as a "nonablative" laser. That means that unlike the resurfacing lasers commonly used to smooth wrinkled and sun-damaged or acne-scarred skin (see pages 183-184), it does not strip off (ablate) the skin. Instead, it works beneath the surface, by emitting a beam that penetrates the epidermis and is absorbed by water in the middle layer of the skin, the dermis. The water heats up, which inflicts an injury to the tissues there, including the sebaceous glands. (A built-in spraying device simultaneously applies a mist of coolant to the skin's surface to reduce pain and discomfort from the heat.) This shrinks the glands, reducing their capacity to produce sebum.

Smoothbeam treatment requires a series of office visits, ranging from three to five treatments, spaced three to four weeks apart. In one of the initial trials, seventeen study subjects (treated for acne on their backs) received a series of four treatments, spaced four weeks apart. Six months after the last treatment, sixteen of them still had complete clearing of their acne lesions.

LOOK OUT FOR PITFALLS

With all acne treatments and the sometimes complex multi-drug regimens they require, the difference between success and failure frequently hinges on what doctors call compliance— that is, whether the patients use the medicines exactly as they are intended to be used in order to get the most out of them.

Dermatologists say these are the most common pitfalls:

- **Using other medications that may conflict with acne treatment.** Different combinations of drugs can produce unwanted side effects or interfere with the activity of one or more of the drugs. That is why doctors always want to know everything you are taking (including herbal remedies or dietary supplements) before they prescribe something new. With acne, you also need to tell your dermatologist about all the things you regularly apply to your skin, such as cosmetics, moisturizers, sunscreens, and over-the-counter acne medicines. Many of them can make your skin overly sensitive to prescription topical agents; often you have to stop using them while on prescription therapy.

- **Doubling up or otherwise exceeding a prescribed dose.** Whether it is an oral medicine that you take by mouth, or a topical one that you apply to your skin, the prescribed amounts are calculated to achieve maximum results with minimal side effects. Don't assume that if a little of something is beneficial, a lot more will be even more effective, or that it will work any faster. It won't. What overdosing *will* do is increase the potential for unpleasant, even dangerous side effects, forcing you to abandon the very remedies you need.

- **Skipping doses—the alternate route to failure.** Swallowing pills or applying topical medicines at regular intervals is essential for maintaining effective levels of any acne medicine in the body and on the skin. British dermatologist and noted acne researcher William Cunliffe has likened acne medication to birth control pills: skip a few doses, and you've lost your protection and are back at square one. This includes keeping up with a maintenance treatment routine once your skin is clear. Never forget, the key to effective acne treatment is prevention. "As long as you have acne-prone skin, you have to keep treating it," warns Alan Shalita. "If you don't, the acne will be back in a month."

Chapter Seven

—◇—

Accutane

ABOUT THE TIME I STARTED writing this book, a friend of mine introduced me to her daughter, a young woman in her mid-twenties who a couple of years earlier had begun to experience severe acne breakouts. We talked for a long time about her various unsuccessful treatments, her despair over the obvious scarring she had experienced, and her growing unhappiness with her dermatologist, who, she reported, could come up with nothing to help her.

"Do you know, he actually wants me to take *Accutane!*" she declared, as appalled as if the doctor had proposed amputation. When I told her that Accutane had been the answer to my prayers, and might well be the answer to hers, she looked at me as if I were insane. "I can't take *Accutane,*" she insisted. "It's just too scary."

Accutane is a very scary drug to many people, and it certainly is not one to be taken lightly. It can cause a number of serious side effects, including severe birth defects in the unborn children of women who become pregnant while using it. Accutane has also been suspected of causing depression or psychotic behavior in some patients.

In recent years, the widely reported suicides of two teenage Accutane patients—one the son of a U.S. congressman, the other a student pilot who crashed his small plane into the side of a Florida office building—focused new attention on the drug's possible psychiatric side effects. This reignited a long-smoldering controversy within the medical community and the Food and Drug Administration as to whether it should be more tightly regulated or even withdrawn from the market entirely.

And yet, for millions of acne patients, Accutane has proved to be a genuine miracle drug in the years since its introduction in 1982. Speaking as one of those patients, I can say that it truly transformed my life. Finding something that actually worked after twenty years of futile effort seemed miraculous in every way to me. Echoing a sentiment common among his fellow dermatologists, leading acne researcher James Leyden has called Accutane "the single most significant advance in acne therapy."

Louisiana's Dr. John Yarborough, a widely respected dermatologic surgeon with decades of experience in treating faces ravaged by acne scars, says, "I truly believe that to my generation of physicians, Accutane is the same sort of miracle drug that penicillin was to that generation of physicians."

HISTORY OF A MIRACLE DRUG

Accutane is the U.S. brand name for the drug isotretinoin, patented by drug manufacturer Roche Pharmaceuticals. In Europe, Canada, and the United Kingdom, it is known as Roaccutane. Roche's patent for isotretinoin expired in 2001, opening the way for competing drug companies to offer generic versions. The first of these rival medicines earned FDA approval in late 2002; versions are now available to the public under the names Amnesteem, Claravis, and Sotret.

Like Retin-A and other topical retinoids used to treat acne, isotretinoin is derived from vitamin A. The difference is that isotretinoin is an oral retinoid, one that is taken by mouth rather than applied to the skin.

Scientists have known for decades about vitamin A's therapeutic effects on the skin. Sometimes called the "anti-infective" vitamin, it plays a key role in maintaining the health of skin cells. However, the body does not readily excrete vitamin A, and taken in large doses it can build up to toxic levels. That is why retinoids used to treat disease often have serious side effects.

In the 1970s, Swiss-based drug giant Hoffmann-La Roche (parent company of the U.S. firm) synthesized a number of different retinoids, trying to come up with safe versions for use on a variety of skin conditions. Among the experimental compounds was one known as 13 cis-retinoic acid. Dermatologist Gary L. Peck, leading a group of researchers at the National Institutes of Health, tried it on fourteen patients (eight men and six women) who had an exceptionally severe and disfiguring form of acne called *acne conglobata*. *Acne conglobata* is acne at its most extreme and uncontrollable; at the time it was regarded by dermatologists as truly hopeless. There was literally no effective means of treating it.

Astoundingly, after four months of taking the new drug, thirteen of the fourteen patients were completely free of the monstrous cysts and nodules that had covered their backs and faces; the remaining patient was not totally clear, but had improved dramatically.

When Peck and his colleagues published their results in 1979, in the *New England Journal of Medicine*, the report caused a sensation among dermatologists. Potential patients who got wind of the new discovery from press accounts of an "acne cure" went wild with hope. Reportedly, one young man was so desperate to obtain Accutane for his girlfriend that he attempted to acquire a supply by holding up the NIH pharmacy at gunpoint.

WHAT IT DOES

Isotretinoin is so dramatically effective against acne because it is the only medicine that effectively fights breakouts on all major fronts. It reduces the size of sebaceous glands, which dramatically curtails sebum production; it decreases the cellular buildup that leads to comedones in sebaceous follicles; it massacres the population of P. acnes bacteria; and it quells inflammation. Most remarkably, the drug's therapeutic effects typically last long after a patient has stopped taking it. Alone among acne medicines, isotretinoin produces lasting beneficial changes in the skin, making it a virtual cure for many acne patients and dramatically lessening symptoms over the long term for almost all others.

The most common side effects of isotretinoin are similar to those produced by overdosing on vitamin A, a condition called "hypervitaminosis A," or vitamin A toxicity. For most people, the symptoms show up in the mucous membranes and the skin. Accutane makes the skin very dry and easily irritated. The single most common side effect—affecting up to 95 percent of all Accutane patients—is excessively dry, cracked lips. Some patients also get dry, irritated eyes (which can be a particular problem for contact lens wearers). Others may develop thinning hair or intermittent headaches. Muscular aches or joint pain may become a problem, particularly for people who tend to be very active or athletic.

More serious side effects are uncommon. They include colitis (an inflammation of the colon's mucous membrane); impaired night vision, which can make it impossible to drive after dark; increased lipid levels in the blood; elevated liver enzymes; and hepatitis. All of these effects are reversible; they typically disappear once the drug is stopped. The one exception is the most serious of all possible consequences: damage to the unborn child if a woman takes the drug while pregnant.

Accutane and Pregnancy

From the beginning, doctors knew that isotretinoin could cause birth defects. All known oral retinoids (including vitamin A itself, if taken in large enough doses) are teratogenic, meaning that they can harm the cells of a developing fetus. The paper that published the results of the original NIH study warned of isotretinoin's possible danger to unborn babies, and Accutane labeling has always carried strong warnings about pregnancy. Over the years, patient advocacy groups and some medical experts, including some staffers at the Food and Drug Administration and the Centers for Disease Control, have called for it to be taken off the market because of the severity of the threat.

The danger cannot be overemphasized. Although not every infant exposed to Accutane in the womb has been born deformed, the risk of birth defects is extremely high, with the greatest danger apparently occurring early in the pregnancy, when even a small amount of the drug—just a few pills—can be devastating.

A woman who becomes pregnant while taking isotretinoin may suffer a miscarriage; an estimated four out of ten pregnancies exposed to Accutane end in spontaneous abortions. For babies that are carried to term, common fetal abnormalities include heart, brain, and central nervous system defects; skull anomalies (children may be born with exceptionally small or asymmetric heads); and facial malformations such as cleft palate. Deformed eyes or ears are also common; some infants who have been exposed to Accutane in the womb are born without ears or other facial features.

Even if they do not have obvious physical deformities, Accutane-exposed babies may be mentally retarded or experience severe developmental difficulties. In one survey of young children whose mothers had taken Accutane while pregnant, more than half of the offspring had IQs of eighty-five or below. This is the IQ range at which youngsters generally require special education; it is also an indication that they may not be able to live independently as adults.

Because of these risks, doctors are extremely cautious when prescribing the drug to any woman of childbearing age, including young teenage girls who may not yet be sexually active, and it has always been sold with forcefully worded labels warning of the dangers. There are no similar precautions for men; isotretinoin has no known impact on sperm cells, and babies fathered by men taking Accutane have shown no ill effects. Similarly, Accutane has no effect on the ovaries and will not jeopardize a woman's chances of having healthy children in the future. The threat is solely to babies in the wombs of expectant mothers.

Tragically, a number of women over the years have become pregnant while taking Accutane. One investigation revealed that some had ignored the warnings or had not been fully informed of the necessary precautions for using the drug. In fact, a graphic symbol designed to reinforce written and verbal admonitions about pregnancy actually backfired in a few cases. Consisting of a slashed-circle (like a do-not-enter traffic sign) superimposed over the silhouette of a pregnant woman, the illustration was evidently misinterpreted by some women to mean that the drug was a contraceptive.

In 2002, Roche and the FDA hammered out a stringent (albeit voluntary) new patient monitoring and education program, called the System to Manage Accutane-Related Teratogenicity, or SMART. (Amnesteem, the first competing version of Accutane, debuted with a similar program called SPIRIT, for System to Prevent Isotretinoin-Related Issues of Teratogenicity.) The goal was to unite doctors, patients, and pharmacists in an all-out effort to prevent women who are already pregnant from taking Accutane and to keep women who are taking the drug from becoming pregnant while on it.

In order to prescribe Accutane, physicians are now asked to register with Roche and sign an agreement saying they understand the drug's risks and that they will follow SMART guidelines for prescribing it. Before they can prescribe Accutane to women (or teenage girls), doctors must first provide counseling about effective pregnancy prevention. They must also have their patients (both male and female) sign a detailed consent form indicating that they are aware of all of the drug's risks.

Before you can receive a prescription for Accutane, you must now have two negative urine or serum pregnancy tests— an initial one for screening, and a second one in the first five days of the menstrual period that occurs immediately before you get your prescription. You must also agree to use two forms of birth control (or avoid intercourse completely) while taking the drug, and for a month afterward. You will then receive a prescription for a single month's supply only. Each month thereafter, before getting a refill prescription, you will have to return to your doctor for another pregnancy test— even if you are not sexually active.

Your doctor will also ask you to register in an ongoing Accutane patient survey conducted by Boston University's Sloan School of Epidemiology. Although registration in the Sloan Survey is voluntary (your doctor cannot deny you a prescription for Accutane if you refuse to sign up), a major goal of the SMART program is to enroll at least 60 percent of all Accutane patients in order to gather more comprehensive data on all of the drug's side effects than has been available thus far.

Each Accutane prescription you receive will be labeled with a bright yellow qualification sticker (available from Roche to physicians who have agreed to comply with the program) to show your pharmacist that you have fulfilled all of the requirements and are, in effect, "qualified" to receive Accutane—i.e., that you are not pregnant, and that you are fully informed of all the risks. For their part, pharmacists will fill only prescriptions bearing the yellow sticker and not take phone orders. They will dispense only one month's supply at a time, and not fill prescriptions more than seven days old.

ACCUTANE AND DEPRESSION

Somewhat ironically, the SMART program debuted at a time when public attention on Accutane was focused not so much on its proven dangers as a teratogen, but on its rare, yet much more controversial association with psychiatric side effects.

While there is a clear cause-and-effect biological connection between isotretinoin and birth defects, a definitive link between the drug and psychiatric problems has thus far been impossible to establish. The principal body of evidence implicating isotretinoin in psychiatric disorders comes from what are known as "Adverse Drug Event Reports." These consist of information sent by physicians to the Food and Drug Administration detailing individual cases in which a given drug produces severe or unexpected side effects.

Between 1982, when Accutane was approved for sale in

the United States, and May 2000, 18.8 percent of the adverse event reports for the drug documented psychiatric problems, most seriously depression and suicide. Over that period, there were twenty-four reported suicides in U.S. patients taking Accutane and those who had recently stopped taking it. The FDA also received reports of 110 Accutane users in the United States who had been hospitalized for depression, attempted suicide, or thoughts of suicide (suicide "ideation," as it is called). During that time there were another 284 reports of Accutane users who were diagnosed with depression but not hospitalized.

Such numbers are extremely small in comparison to the millions of people who have uneventfully taken Accutane since 1982, and several large epidemiological studies have found that the rates of suicide and depression among Accutane patients are no greater (indeed, in the case of suicide, it is actually dramatically less) than among the general population as a whole.

But while psychiatric side effects may be rare, they remain a serious concern to the FDA and to doctors who prescribe the drug. "I think, and this is just speculation, that there may be a small subset of patients who have some sort of chemical abnormality or difference that makes them susceptible to direct depression as a result of the drug," says SUNY's Alan Shalita, who has treated thousands of patients with Accutane, without seeing any of them suffer from severe psychiatric side effects. "I believe that's an infinitesimally small percent of the population, but several of my colleagues have seen people who have had depression with Accutane, and it's the kind of problem that dermatologists should be aware of and talk to their patients about."

The medication guide that patients now receive with their prescriptions for Accutane contains a checklist of warning signs that urges you to stop taking the drug and immediately contact your doctor if you start to feel sad or have crying spells, lose interest in your usual activities, experience changes in your normal sleep patterns, become more irritable than usual, lose your appetite, become unusually tired, have trouble concentrating, withdraw from family and friends, or start having thoughts about hurting yourself or committing suicide.

WHO SHOULD TAKE ACCUTANE

Accutane is approved by the Food and Drug Administration for "severe recalcitrant nodular acne" that has proved unresponsive to all other therapies. The prescribing information characterizes this type of acne specifically as inflamed nodules or cysts that are lodged deep within the skin and that may be bleeding or pus-filled. It also sternly notes that "'severe' by definition means 'many' as opposed to 'few or several' nodules."

When Accutane first came on the market, most dermatologists adhered closely to those guidelines (what are called "indications"). I vividly, in fact, bitterly, recall visiting a succession of dermatologists during those early years and being repeatedly told that my so-called moderate acne was "not serious enough" for Accutane, even though nothing else had ever worked for me, and I was steadily acquiring obvious acne scars. It took several years before I finally found a doctor who agreed that Accutane was appropriate for me. (Thank you, Dr. Castillo!)

Today, most acne-savvy dermatologists would consider me to have been an Accutane candidate from the start. In the years since isotretinoin was introduced, the trend in prescribing has been a steady expansion of the indications to include relatively moderate acne that has failed over time to respond to conventional treatment such as antibiotics and topical retinoids—just like my skin in the mid-1980s, with its few but persistent pimples and periodic flares of large, unsightly nodules.

This, of course, is precisely the kind of acne that plagues many adult women, noted Dr. William J. Cunliffe, of England's University of Leeds, at a meeting of the World Congress of Dermatology in 2002. "At thirty-five, they may have had acne for twenty years. You can try treating it conventionally with topical therapy, but often these patients are a little tired of such therapy."

Philadelphia's Dr. Albert Kligman agrees. "I used to say treat postadolescent acne in women the same way you treat acne in other cases. But I underestimated the difficulty. Those crops of deep lesions that a lot of women get can go on for months without anything happening. And women don't want to be left hanging around for months without seeing any progress. So my view now is to go right to the top and bomb it with Accutane. Because my experience has been that treating this kind of acne the way you treat ordinary, adolescent acne is a mistake. It's too difficult and it takes too long."

Dermatologists today are also prompt to consider Accutane for any acne patient who is scarring, or who has a tendency to scar, whatever the severity of the disease, and for those who are suffering from significant emotional distress, even if their acne is relatively mild. An international survey published in 1997 showed that dermatologists around the world now use isotretinoin for these broader indications.

None of this means that any dermatologist will necessarily give you Accutane right off the bat. "For a lot of us, deciding when to use Accutane is part of the art of treating acne," says acne specialist Dr. Diane Berson, adjunct assistant professor of dermatology at New York University. "If the patient is responding, even slowly, to other medication, I usually wait and give it a chance."

TAKING ACCUTANE

Just how much of a chance your doctor will give other medicines to work before turning to Accutane depends on his or her individual judgment and experience. It could be anywhere from a few months to a year; there are no hard and fast rules. There is, however, one reason in particular that experienced acne doctors do not usually immediately write an Accutane prescription even for someone whose acne seems to be crying out for it: the fear of inciting an acne flare.

As sometimes happens with topical retinoids, isotretinoin may make acne worse before it makes it better. In some cases it can become horrendously worse, producing out-of-control inflammatory lesions that can leave terrible scars. The cause is apparently isotretinoin's dramatic effect on sebum production; the drug virtually shuts down the oil glands, starving out *P. acnes* bacteria. If there are a lot of bacteria, their mass death by famine produces a sudden flood of inflammatory chemicals that can set off an explosion of both inflamed and previously noninflamed lesions. The danger is particularly acute for a patient with many large, noninflamed, closed comedones (so-called "macrocomedones") or persistent secondary comedones lingering deep in the skin.

Dermatologists who are experienced in prescribing Accutane employ several strategies to head off flares. The first step is to get inflammation as much under control as possible with a pre-Accutane course of oral antibiotics or steroids. Doctors may also surgically extract or drain large closed comedones to ensure that they don't erupt into destructive inflamed lesions. The Accutane is then gradually introduced at a very low dose, minimizing the potential for side effects while gradually working up over a period of weeks to the optimal daily amount. Acne experts stress that it is crucial to *never* start at the maximum dose.

Just as there are no stringent rules about who should be taking isotretinoin and when any individual should start, there are also no precise guidelines for determining the precise amount that is best for any individual patient. Experience has shown that for most people on Accutane, it takes a total cumulative dose of about 120 milligrams per kilogram of the patient's body weight to clear up the acne and effect prolonged changes in the skin.

Generally speaking, there are two schools of thought about how best to arrive at that figure: the high-dose school and the low-dose school.

The amount of isotretinoin you take each day is calculated according to your weight. The standard rule of thumb is 1 milligram per kilogram of body weight per day (after the initial break-in period at a much lower dose). For most women, this translates to a relatively rapid four-month (or thereabouts) course of treatment.

This is the most common approach—the "high-dose" school. It is the method most frequently employed in the United States. Doctors are particularly inclined to use it for women, in order to expose the fewest menstrual cycles possible to the drug and thus reduce the risk of an unintended pregnancy. It also means that a patient will only have to put up with any unpleasant side effects that might occur for just a few months.

On the other hand, fans of the "low-dose" method (more common in Europe and Great Britain) point out that taking a much lower than average daily dose, or an intermittent one (only a few pills a week), for a longer period of time, tends to produce far fewer side effects in the first place—although, be aware, it does *not* reduce the risks associated with pregnancy. According to Cunliffe, low-dose Accutane treatment is often an excellent choice for women with mild acne, or whose acne may be under control, but who are still plagued with excessively oily skin. "These patients get great results on low-dose, intermittent therapy, and with virtually no side effects."

"Americans are always pushing the high dose," notes Germany's Professor Gerd Plewig. "But we like to use the ultra-low dose. It is very helpful for these women, and many of them have wonderful skin for a long time after. We have done this for many years, and we think it is much better for the patient. Usually after a year, I tell them we should stop, but they never want to. They become addicted."

Whatever regimen a patient is on, all other prescription and OTC acne medicines are stopped while on Accutane. Doctors also advise against taking supplemental vitamin A and aspirin (which may make a patient more vulnerable to damage to the mucous membranes). They recommend gentle cleansers and non-comedogenic moisturizers to counter any facial dryness and oil-free broad-spectrum sunscreens during the day.

Dermatologists also recommend highly emollient lip ointments to deal with dry lips. A company called Summers Laboratory (www.sumlab.com) makes a special lip balm, Accu-soothe, specifically for the excessively dry lips of Accutane patients; it also contains sunscreen. Other very greasy lip ointments, or plain Vaseline, also work well; waxy lip balms generally are not sufficiently emollient to help.

By shutting down the sebaceous glands, Accutane makes the skin more vulnerable to injury; it does not heal as quickly and may produce more significant scars if wounded. So patients are usually advised to avoid any cosmetic or other elective surgery for at least six months after taking Accutane. Some dermatologic surgeons recommend waiting as long as two years before undergoing laser resurfacing, deep chemical peels, or dermabrasion.

"It is very important to warn patients about increased skin fragility," cautions Berson. "A lot of women who have acne are also hirsute, and a lot of them get waxed to remove the hairs from their face. And we've seen patients who've developed erosions and blistering at the areas where they've been waxed. So women should be advised to either avoid waxing if they are taking the drug, or to first do a small test site to make sure they're not prone to injury."

WHAT IF IT DOESN'T WORK?
ISOTRETINOIN-"RESISTANT" ACNE

Doctors who prescribe Accutane are careful to point out that it is not a true "cure" for acne; indeed, ads for the drug describe its effects as "prolonged remission." Even so it is a virtual cure for many. Surveys of Accutane patients show that it eliminates or greatly reduces severe acne in around 80 percent of the patients who take it. After a course of treatment, sebum production gradually returns to around its original, pretreatment levels. But for the majority of patients, this does not bring on new waves of serious acne.

About 17 percent of Accutane cases require a second course of the drug, typically after a six-month hiatus. Patients whose acne returns after that are generally regarded as having "failed."

There are a number of possible reasons for Accutane failure. An increasingly troubling one to dermatologists is inappropriate use. "Isotretinoin should really only be prescribed by doctors who are experienced and competent in the diagnosis and treatment of severe recalcitrant acne and who are very familiar with the use of retinoids," says Berson.

In a 2002 American Academy of Dermatology talk on isotretinoin resistance, Dr. Guy Webster, vice chair of the Department of Dermatology at Philadelphia's Jefferson Medical College, noted that in recent years half of the severe acne patients referred to his department for evaluation have come from nondermatologists who have given Accutane a try and been unsuccessful in getting their patients better.

According to Webster, some of those patients should not even have been given Accutane in the first place because they did not actually have acne; their physicians had misdiagnosed one of the many acne-like disorders.

But the chief cause of true isotretinoin failure is inadequate dosage—not using the right dose long enough. Sometimes other drugs may interfere with Accutane; seizure medication such as Dilantin may increase sebaceous gland output and counteract the effects of Accutane. Sometimes patients, for some reason, do not absorb retinoids well, blunting their effect. For women, one of the most common causes of all is some kind of hormonal irregularity—an idiosyncrasy that keeps the sebaceous glands pumping despite the Accutane. For these patients, the logical next step is an investigation of the hormonal factors at work on their skin.

Chapter Eight

———◦———

Hormones and Hormonal Treatment

INEVITABLY, ALMOST ANY DISCUSSION about acne and women comes down to hormones. After all, it is hormones and their control over sebaceous follicles that bring on acne in the first place. And hormonal influences are clearly responsible for the fact that there are so many more adult women than adult men with acne. Acne-prone men typically experience only one major acne-inciting hormonal event—puberty, when testosterone soars and pimples erupt. Then, for most males, acne dies down. But for acne-prone women, puberty is only the beginning of a lifetime of significant hormonal incidents—menstruation, ovulation, pregnancy, birth, lactation, menopause—that can all trigger or exacerbate breakouts.

Hormones are intrinsically complex, and the science of endocrinology (the study of hormones) is still a relatively new field. Understandably, many dermatologists—experts in skin, not the endocrine system—are wary of embarking on hormonal therapy for their acne patients. Yet it has become increasingly clear that for numerous women with persistent acne that defies all conventional treatments, pinning down a hormonal cause and addressing it may be the only means of controlling it. According to one estimate, as many as 60 percent of women suffering from adult-onset acne or worsening acne in adulthood either do not respond well to conventional therapy, or build up a tolerance to frequently used medicines.

"I'm really hot on using hormones for females with adult acne," says Dr. Wilma Bergfeld, head of Dermopathology and Clinical Research at Ohio's Cleveland Clinic, and an authority on hormonal disorders of the skin. "I see a lot of women with stubborn acne in my practice, and their biggest problem is that their physician has given them the usual acne therapies, but hasn't gone after the source of the problem—which many times is hormonal. And for those women, until you've got the hormones under control, the acne keeps coming back. My practice is to go after the cause. And when I do that, I can clear them up."

ACNE AND THE HORMONAL BALLET

Altogether, more than two hundred hormones and hormone-like substances direct and regulate every system and function in our bodies. These chemical messengers travel via the blood-stream to far-flung parts of the body where they latch on to cells (called targets) and deliver their orders.

There isn't an organ that isn't affected by hormonal shifts and balances, and the whole system of hormone production and deployment comprises a seemingly infinite number of variations. Teasing apart the various possible interactions to pin down precisely how any hormone or group of hormones affects any one organ is a herculean task. Figuring out the complex hormonal influences involved in acne is no exception.

The sebaceous follicles, where acne occurs, are controlled by the family of hormones known as androgens, which are manufactured in the ovaries and the adrenal glands. (The androgens in turn are part of an even larger extended family—

the steroids, which also include estrogen and progesterone, the hormones that regulate female reproductive functions.)

The androgen most directly implicated in making your skin break out is testosterone. Although women have only about one tenth as much testosterone as men, it is nonetheless the most abundant androgen found in healthy women, and it serves a number of functions, including acting on androgen receptor sites in muscles to promote muscle growth—what is known as the anabolic effect.

A "carrier" protein called sex hormone binding globulin (SHBG), produced by the liver, helps transport androgens through the body. SHBG can be a critical factor in acne, because it determines how much of the androgens in your bloodstream actually reach their targets in the skin; androgens bound to SHBG are less able to interact with target tissues than when they are floating free in the circulatory system.

The androgens are master shape-shifters. Depending on where they are in the body and what receptor cells happen to be nearby, any of them can be converted into testosterone. (Some researchers speculate that this chameleon-like ability may be a control mechanism to ensure that cells with testosterone receptors are always assured of an adequate supply, without the body having to maintain huge amounts of testosterone in the blood where it might make its way to places it is not needed and produce undesirable side effects.)

About 25 percent of the testosterone that ultimately reaches the skin comes directly from the ovaries. All of the rest is created on the spot, from other, weaker androgens circulating in the blood. In the skin, an enzyme called 5-alpha reductase effects yet a final transformation: It turns testosterone into an even more potent version of itself, called dihydrotestosterone (DHT).

DHT is the switch that turns on the sebaceous gland, stimulating it to produce acne-fueling sebum. In fact, DHT acts on the entire pilosebaceous unit—the hair follicle as well as the sebaceous gland. So, in addition to stimulating oil production, it also affects hair growth. This is why acne in women sometimes comes hand in hand with hair loss or excessive hair growth (hirsutism) in typically male patterns: on the face, the back, the chest, the groin. Sometimes, women will experience all of these symptoms at once: male pattern baldness, hirsutism, and acne. They are all known as "androgen-dependent" diseases, and DHT has a hand in each.

HORMONAL FACTORS THAT AFFECT ACNE

Anything that affects androgen production by either the adrenal glands or the ovaries can potentially affect acne-prone skin. For example, stress, which stimulates the adrenals, can increase androgen production and may lead to an acne flare.

There are many such influences on androgen production, from natural hormonal events like menstruation, to the activities of other endocrine glands such as the pituitary, which governs both the adrenals and the ovaries. The picture may be further complicated by hormones that come from outside your body. Going on the Pill or stopping it, beginning or ending hormone replacement therapy, or taking certain dietary supplements can all affect the hormones that affect your skin. The presence of hormones or hormone-like substances in the environment and in foods may also influence androgen production in your body.

For acne-prone women, even minor hormonal imbalances may show up on the skin as pimples. And even if your hormonal levels fall in the normal range, you may suffer from what is known as "end organ hyperresponsiveness." In other words, you may not have unusually high androgen levels, but your skin overreacts to the normal androgens that are there.

You may also have overactive androgen receptors in your skin; in which case, whenever any testosterone reaches the follicles, your hyped-up receptors will grab more than their share. Or, the fault may lie with the testosterone-converting enzyme, 5-alpha reductase. Researchers suspect that 5-alpha reductase may be more abundant or more active in women with acne than in those with clear skin.

ACNE AND YOUR NORMAL HORMONAL LIFE

Premenstrual Flares

The phenomenon of premenstrual acne is so common that many women take it for granted. But despite the fact that millions of women experience these clockwork-like flares every month, there has been virtually no scientific research to investigate it, much less explain it. It wasn't until 2001 that the first large-scale study ever of premenstrual acne was published. It confirmed, in a survey of 400 women, that, yes (duh!), acne did flare for many women prior to menstruation, with nearly half experiencing premenstrual breakouts of some kind. It also indicated that premenstrual acne is somewhat more likely to occur in older women, although the reasons are not clear.

In most cases, premenstrual acne lesions appear after ovulation and before menses. Typically several large, tender inflamed nodules will pop up about a week before menstruation, preceding other premenstrual symptoms such as water retention, breast tenderness, or mood changes by several days. Apparently, they arise from invisible, closed comedones that are already lurking in the skin.

But the mechanism remains unknown. One possible explanation: At midcycle, the pituitary gland releases what is known as luteinizing hormone (or LH), which stimulates the ovaries. This results in both ovulation and a spurt of increased androgen production. This in turn may lead to more testosterone in the skin, inciting accelerated sebaceous gland activity, which stimulates or exacerbates breakouts.

Pregnancy and Lactation

Pregnancy's effect on acne-prone skin is even more difficult to pin down. Evidently, pregnancy does have an impact on sebaceous glands; for example, those around the nipple enlarge during gestation, appearing as small brown papules. But the role of pregnancy on any individual woman's acne is completely unpredictable. For some, breakouts disappear entirely; for others, acne appears for the first time.

Medical science does not yet have a good explanation in either case, although there is one possible mechanism at work on women whose acne improves during pregnancy: the increase in estrogen levels, which peak in the third trimester. In the skin, estrogen competes with testosterone for the same receptor sites. Essentially that means that if the body has additional estrogen, more of it will attach to androgen receptors in the skin, thus shouldering out acne-stimulating testosterone.

Conversely, estrogen levels fall off after delivery. This can lead to acne or temporary hair loss two to four months later, as levels of testosterone rise relative to the amount of competing estrogen.

Perimenopause and Menopause

During perimenopause, the span of time preceding menopause, a woman's ovaries gradually produce less estrogen. Androgen production is higher in comparison, which creates an imbalance that can lead to excess testosterone at the skin receptor sites—and perimenopausal acne.

Androgen production as a whole declines after menopause, which is when the ovaries stop producing estrogen altogether. But you can still have acne from excess androgens as long as your ovaries are still putting out testosterone, which gradually tapers away over the decade following menopause.

"Most women who have acne after menopause are in the category of androgen excess," explains Bergfeld. "Androgen excess is something you see most often in younger women, but you also get a subset at menopause. There are cells in the ovaries and the adrenals which can overproduce androgens in the menopausal years—a sudden spontaneous overgrowth of certain tissues that express androgens, and that can keep giving you acne."

Menopausal women on hormone replacement therapy containing testosterone may also get acne—or show other signs of androgen excess such as hirsutism or male-pattern baldness.

MEDICAL CONDITIONS THAT CAN LEAD TO HORMONAL ACNE

Polycystic Ovary Syndrome

One of the most common causes of androgen excess in women is a condition called polycystic ovary syndrome (PCOS), in which small noncancerous cysts in the ovaries produce abnormal levels of androgens.

Most ovarian cysts are an abnormal consequence of normal cyclical changes. Each month, as a woman ovulates, an egg is released from the ovary, leaving behind a ruptured follicle that briefly transforms into a small, independent organ—the corpus luteum. The corpus luteum pumps out the hormone progesterone, which signals the uterus to prepare to receive a fertilized egg, marking the start of pregnancy. If no pregnancy occurs, the corpus luteum is programmed to self-destruct and shut down progesterone production.

But sometimes, instead of dying, the corpus luteum evolves into a cyst that continues to make progesterone. Multiple cysts create hormonal havoc by altering hormonal balance. As well as acne, the symptoms may include irregular or no menstrual periods, high blood pressure, hair loss, hirsutism, infertility, weight gain, and diabetes or insulin resistance.

PCOS is very common; to one degree or another it affects as many as one out of ten women of childbearing age in the United States. And, according to one estimate, close to 40 percent of all adult women with acne have some form of PCOS.

Insulin Resistance

About half of all women with PCOS are overweight—which reduces their cells' sensitivity to insulin and may cause insulin resistance, a condition which in itself can contribute to acne. Insulin, produced by the pancreas, is the hormone responsible for transferring sugar in the blood (glucose) into the body's cells, to be used as fuel. In other words, insulin is the key that unlocks the cells so they can receive glucose.

Insulin resistance is a condition in which cells become insensitive or nonreactive to the insulin "key"; they no longer allow it to "unlock" them normally and let glucose in. As a result, both insulin levels and glucose levels in the blood rise.

High levels of insulin in the blood, in turn, overwhelm receptors on the ovaries, stimulating them to increase their production of androgens. High levels of insulin can also lead to lower-than-normal levels of sex hormone binding globulin

(SHBG), the testosterone carrier. As a result, women with insulin resistance may have more free testosterone in their blood, available to reach the sebaceous follicles and cause acne—not to mention all of the other symptoms of excess testosterone.

Ovarian or Adrenal Tumors

Benign or malignant tumors on either the ovaries or the adrenal glands may also produce excess testosterone. This is very rare, but doctors may suspect it if a woman very suddenly starts breaking out with acne and showing other signs (hirsutism, male pattern baldness, voice changes, weight gain) that suggest high testosterone levels. Another possible sign of a tumor is if acne persists even despite hormonal therapies.

Adrenal Disorders

A condition called congenital adrenal hyperplasia (CAH) is an inherited disorder that leads to hyperactivity of the adrenal glands and increased androgen levels in the blood. Classic CAH is a very serious disease that is usually diagnosed in childhood. Another form, called nonclassic or adult-onset congenital adrenal hyperplasia, is sometimes the cause of elevated androgens and hormonal acne. In another adrenal condition, called Cushing's syndrome, the adrenal glands may release too much of an androgen called dehydroepiandrosterone sulfate (DHEA-S), which may be transformed into testosterone at the skin—and can lead to acne.

DECIDING ON HORMONAL TREATMENT

Even if a woman has hormonally influenced acne, most doctors will stick with conventional therapy if it seems to be working. But if your acne does not respond to conventional treatment, or if you have acne combined with other worrisome signs of hormonal irregularity (menstrual problems, excess body hair, a recent sudden increase in skin oiliness, breakouts or hair on the jawline, or insulin resistance), your doctor may order a series of tests to pin down a hormonal cause. These will include blood tests to check different androgen levels, and perhaps also the levels of sex hormone binding globulin and pituitary hormones that control the ovaries and the adrenal glands. Diagnostic tests may also include a pelvic ultrasound to check for cysts or tumors on the ovaries and adrenal glands, and a check of glucose and insulin levels.

Hormonal therapy for acne is aimed at reducing sebum in the skin, thus choking off the fuel that nourishes the acne flame. In general, there are three ways that drugs can be used to accomplish this:

- by curtailing the production of androgens at their source (either the ovaries or the adrenal glands)

- by blocking androgen receptors in the skin itself

- by inhibiting the activity of the enzyme 5-alpha reductase, which converts testosterone in the skin into the more potent, sebaceous gland–stimulating hormone DHT

Because these are all systemic therapies that act on other organs as well as the skin, a dermatologist will often work with a gynecologist or endocrinologist to prescribe the most appropriate treatment and to monitor its effects, especially in women over the age of forty or those who are smokers.

DRUGS THAT REDUCE
ANDROGEN PRODUCTION

The most common hormonal treatment for acne is the oral contraceptive pill, which blocks androgen production at its source. While there are other drugs that also act on the ovaries and the adrenal glands to reduce androgen output, they are generally used only to treat diseases that affect those organs, and would not be used for acne unless it was a result of one of those conditions.

Birth Control Pills *(Ortho Tri-Cyclen, Estrostep,*
   Alesse, Yasmin, others)
Birth control pills work by suppressing the pituitary hormones (called gonadotropins) that stimulate the ovaries. Suppressing gonadotropins suppresses the ovaries, which in turn prevents ovulation and decreases normal ovarian hormonal output.

   Oral contraceptives act in two ways to reduce sebum and improve acne: By suppressing the ovaries (in order to prevent ovulation), they simultaneously cut down on androgen production. They also stimulate the production of sex hormone binding globulin (SHBG), the carrier protein that latches on to circulating androgens; this, in effect, "soaks up" free testosterone in the blood, further reducing the amount that can reach your skin to trigger acne outbreaks.

   The birth control pills used for treating acne are combination pills. They contain estrogen (in a form called ethinyl estradiol) combined with the hormone progestin, a synthetic form of progesterone, which normalizes menstruation. Because some (usually older) forms of progestin encourage the release of androgens, oral contraceptives containing those are called "androgen dominant" contraceptives; early formulations of the Pill used this type of progestin, and they typically made acne worse.

Most oral contraceptives in use today contain second- or third-generation progestins that are deemed far less androgenic than their predecessors. (On the other hand, the injectable contraceptive Depo-Provera and the contraceptive implant Norplant each contains a potentially androgenic progestin that may aggravate breakouts.)

Ortho Tri-Cyclen, the first birth control pill approved by the FDA to treat acne, uses a synthetic progestin called norgestimate; Estrostep, also FDA-approved for acne, contains one called norethindrone. Alesse, another oral contraceptive frequently prescribed for acne patients, contains levonorgestrel. Yasmin, yet another contraceptive promoted for acne patients, contains drospirenone, which is not a progestin but a chemical that acts to block androgen receptors.

Because they all act on the ovaries, birth control pills can be particularly helpful for women whose acne is associated with polycystic ovary syndrome or for those with premenstrual flares. But they are not a cure for acne. They only modestly reduce oil production and the resulting changes in your acne will be slow. It will probably take about two cycles before your sebum production begins to decrease, and as many as five cycles to see real improvement in the skin. Some women experience acne flares during the first couple of cycles. Most doctors recommend that birth control pills used to treat acne be used in combination with other acne drugs such as topical retinoids and antibiotics. Birth control pills can also be used with other hormonal therapies, in particular, androgen receptor blockers such as spironolactone (discussed below).

Patients whose acne improves while on the Pill will sometimes begin to worsen after about a year of therapy, possibly due to a feedback effect: The body eventually realizes that the testosterone levels are a little lower than nature intends them to be, so it steps up testosterone production—which may stimulate new breakouts. The Pill can also set you up for a boomerang effect down the road when you eventually go off it. Deprived of the Pill's synthetic estrogen, the body suddenly has far less estrogen to compete with the testosterone at the skin's receptor sites, and this may trigger a dramatic acne flare.

Corticosteroids *(Prednisone, Dexamethasone)*

Oral corticosteriods, which are synthetic hormones similar to natural androgens, act on the adrenal glands to reduce their output of androgens. Because of their many side effects, they are generally not used to treat acne, although sometimes they may be prescribed for women whose acne is triggered by late-onset adrenal hyperplasia, a condition which causes the adrenal glands to become more active.

ANTI-ANDROGENS

The anti-androgens are drugs that block testosterone at the hormone receptor level, ensuring that the oil-stimulating androgens can't act in the skin to produce extra sebum. This makes them a particularly good choice for women whose acne may stem not from excess testosterone, but from skin that is more than normally sensitive to its effects. Anti-androgen drugs cannot be taken during pregnancy, because they have feminizing effects on male fetuses.

Spironolactone *(Aldactone, Alatone)*

Spironolactone is the most common anti-androgen prescribed for acne. It has been used for over thirty years as a diuretic to treat high blood pressure and liver and kidney disorders. It works by blocking androgen receptors in order to inhibit the adrenal hormone aldosterone, which regulates sodium and

potassium levels in the body. By also blocking androgen receptors in the skin, it coincidentally blocks testosterone and
sebum-stimulating DHT. Spironolactone also inhibits the
activity of the 5-alpha reductase enzyme and decreases some
androgen production in both the ovaries and the adrenal
glands.

Spironolactone can be effectively used in low doses to treat
acne, in conjunction with other acne medication. In order to
reduce side effects (including breast tenderness and menstrual
irregularities), it is usually given in conjunction with oral contraceptives. Its effects on the skin are typically apparent in two
to three months

Because it promotes excretion of sodium and water from
the kidneys and causes the body to retain potassium, you
should not take supplemental potassium or use salt substitutes
if you are on spironolactone. If you are taking ACE inhibitors
or other medicines for a heart condition, your doctor will have
to monitor the levels of those drugs if you begin taking
spironolactone.

Cyproterone acetate (Diane, Dianette)

Another androgen blocker, called cyproterone acetate, is not
available in the United States, but is frequently used in
Canada and Europe as an acne treatment. It is used worldwide
in low doses as the progestin component in oral contraceptives
(Diane, Dianette); this is the form in which it is typically given
to women acne patients.

Flutamide (Euflex, Eulexin)

Flutamide is an androgen receptor blocker that is sometimes
prescribed as an alternative to spironolactone. It is approved
for the treatment of prostate cancer in men (it reduces androgen stimulation of cancerous prostate tissue), and is some-

times prescribed in combination with oral contraceptives for the treatment of acne or excess hair in women. Because it can affect the liver, patients taking it must be monitored for liver function.

5-ALPHA REDUCTASE INHIBITORS

Finasteride *(Propecia, Proscar)*
Widely prescribed as a hair-loss treatment for men (and sometimes for post-menopausal women), finasteride blocks the activity of the enzyme 5-alpha reductase, to inhibit androgen uptake by the hair follicles; this can reduce both hair loss and acne. Finasteride also blocks conversion of testosterone into DHT, the sebum stimulator. But the drug cannot be used by women of childbearing age, because it can cause defects in a male baby's genitalia if the mother takes it when pregnant. Finasteride is so potent that pregnant women are cautioned not even to touch the tablets.

Chapter Nine

———◇———

Herbs, Homeopathy, and Other Alternatives

ONE OF THE FASTEST-GROWING TRENDS in American medicine today is the use of complementary and alternative medicine, sometimes called CAM. Between 1990 and 1997, the number of patient visits to various alternative practitioners in the United States increased from 427 million to 629 million. By 2001, in a variety of health-care practices ranging from acupuncture to homeopathy to massage therapy to traditional Eastern medicine, the United States had 167,300 licensed alternative professional and 221,900 lay practitioners. All told, U.S. consumers spent an estimated $29 billion on alternative therapies that year.

People with skin conditions appear particularly eager to seek out nonconventional medical care. A 1994 survey suggested that 86 percent of all Americans who turned to alternative medicine did so for skin problems.

Certainly, anyone interested in alternative therapy for acne can pick and choose from a wealth of potential remedies, many drawn from centuries of Chinese, Indian, Native American, and European tradition. A host of other options are rooted in the belief that clear skin reflects inner health, which is achieved through holistic regimens that treat the whole person instead of medicating the visibly blemished skin.

But while many alternative acne treatments are backed by a considerable body of lore and have a long history of use, they also have a long history of failure. Indeed, whether it's downing brewer's yeast, shunning dairy products, or applying herbal astringents, most acne patients have tried their share of unconventional treatments over the years, and to little avail.

"You know, it really is a misconception that acne can be cured with a holistic regimen such as diet, herbs, water purification, or acupuncture," says Mount Sinai's Dr. Susan Bershad. "As a general rule, acne does not respond to alternative therapy. As a general rule. There may be some exceptions. But you have to remember that acne is a medical condition, and, on the whole, it really does require medical treatment."

Alternative practitioners, on the other hand, point out that many herbal and other nonconventional remedies for acne do, in fact, have medicinal properties (antiseptic, exfoliating, anti-inflammatory, or hormonal effects) that are very similar to those of conventional acne medicines. And while they may be slower acting and less predictable than the recognized medical therapies, they may also produce fewer undesirable side effects. At the very least, alternative remedies can be valuable adjunctive partners to the more familiar weapons of conventional treatment.

"I practice complementary medicine, so I use a number of different types of things," says Dr. Alan Dattner, one of dermatology's best known and most outspoken proponents of alternative and integrative medicine. In his New York practice, Dattner draws from such diverse techniques as Chinese tongue diagnosis, Ayurvedic therapy from ancient India, herbal medicine, and nutritional modification. But that is not to say he has abandoned the war chest of conventional dermatology. Complementary medicine means using one to complement the other.

"If a woman comes in with cystic acne, I'm going to use antibiotics, because I don't want her to scar, and I'll do whatever it takes to stop it quickly. But at the same time, I'm going to work very hard to figure out how not to need the antibiotics, and make sure I don't have to keep her on the antibiotics for very long."

A NEW LOOK AT DIET

For Dattner, and many other practitioners of complementary dermatology, nutritional therapy ranks high on the list of acne treatments. This flies in the face of research dating back more than forty years that has consistently failed to establish convincing links between acne and diet. In 1969, young acne researchers James Fulton and Gerd Plewig, working with Dr. Albert Kligman at the University of Pennsylvania, published the results of a study in which they fed different groups of acne patients widely differing amounts of chocolate and demonstrated that the long-maligned confection did not either cause or worsen acne. That fabled experiment was followed in turn by tests of numerous other foods suspected of producing breakouts. "And nobody could ever demonstrate they caused acne," says acne expert Dr. Alan Shalita. "Years ago, the University of Missouri tested all of those foods that were commonly believed to make acne worse—dairy foods, sodas, all that stuff—and it turned out that they just didn't."

Today, it is conventional dermatologic wisdom that short of near-starvation (consuming less than a thousand calories a day suppresses sebaceous gland activity), diet plays little or no role in acne. Or, as Kligman puts it, "The sebaceous gland doesn't give a *damn* what you eat!"

Nonetheless, researchers taking a new look at diet today speculate that while the sebaceous glands—which do not excrete dietary fat—may not themselves react directly to the foods you eat, the hormonal mechanisms that control them almost certainly do. As may the potent inflammatory mechanisms that cause so much damage when an acne lesion blows up into an angry red pimple.

In 2002, researchers from the University of Colorado examined the diet of two aboriginal and acne-free populations, the Kiavan Islanders from Papua New Guinea and a tribe of Ache hunter-gatherers from Paraguay. A resulting paper (which was met with widespread skepticism from acne experts) concluded that both groups owed their notably clear complexions to primitive diets free of processed breads, sugars, and cereals. Previous research had shown that when similar tribespeople adopted a Western diet, acne followed. Chief researcher Loren Cordain, a professor of health and exercise science, hypothesized that refined carbohydrates such as sugars and starches cause the body to produce high levels of insulin, creating a hormonal imbalance, which (among other ill effects) can cause an excess of acne-provoking androgens.

Cordain recommends a diet low in sugars and starches, avoiding high-glycemic foods such as bread, potatoes, and sugary desserts, which can all raise blood sugar and trigger high insulin production. Low-glycemic foods favored by Cordain, such as meats, green vegetables, and high-fiber bran products, are less likely to raise insulin levels and create the internal climate that can lead to acne.

"I think people are finding more and more problems with these high-glycemic diets," observes Dattner. "And they may affect acne not just because high carbohydrates raise insulin levels, but also because they release pro-inflammatory chemicals, which add to the problems with inflammation."

Dermatologist Nicholas Perricone, best-selling author of *The Wrinkle Cure* and *The Perricone Prescription*, also indicts inflammation-provoking foods as a major aggravating factor in acne. Perricone believes that inflammation, exacerbated by sugar and other refined carbohydrates, accelerates aging, leading to wrinkles and other age-related conditions—and causes acne. In his book *The Acne Prescription*, he advises acne patients to avoid pro-inflammatory foods. "Basically, that's sugar, or anything that can be rapidly converted to sugar and has a high glycemic index," he says. He proposes instead an "anti-inflammatory" diet high in omega-3 essential fatty acids (found in cold-water fish, especially salmon, some nuts, and olive oil), combined with antioxidant and anti-inflammatory nutritional supplements and topical treatments.

"Acne is an inflammatory disease, and you have to address its inflammatory component," argues Perricone. "And if you can control your blood sugar and your insulin, you can keep inflammation way down. So when people are on an anti-inflammatory diet, their acne improves."

As well as avoiding high-glycemic, inflammation-provoking foods, Alan Dattner also often recommends a dairy-free or low dairy diet for acne patients. "Dairy is one of the most common causes of food allergies, and if you are allergic to dairy components, like casein, it can cause inflammation and other problems in the follicle that can aggravate acne," he explains. "Also, milk contains hormones. About 80 percent of the cows that give milk are pregnant, so you have a lot of progesterone-like hormones in milk. That can affect the androgens that act on sebaceous glands. Plus, nowadays they've thrown in bovine growth hormone, too, and we don't even know what *that* does. The bottom line with dairy foods is that you're providing a hormonal climate that can promote acne."

That's not to say that dairy products necessarily cause or aggravate acne in everyone. Or that eliminating them will always make it go away.

"When you're dealing with a multifactorial problem like acne, it's always hard to get to the bottom of it," says Dattner. "Nature doesn't give up her secrets that easily. But, if a woman has acne, and if she's drinking milk two or three times a day, and she's eating a lot of cheese and other dairy products of all kinds, I think somewhere along the line, before she takes Accutane, or spends two years on tetracycline, it's appropriate to ask, 'What would an elimination diet do?' "

Dattner adds that he often tells acne patients that their breakouts are analogous to a car's oil meter, a visible gauge issuing a warning that something is out of whack. "So just destroying the gauge with antibiotics or covering it with makeup may not be sufficient. I'm not saying don't use those things. I'm just saying that if you see a problem like acne, you should also start questioning what is going on with your life and your diet."

NUTRITIONAL SUPPLEMENTS

Vitamins and minerals are vital to skin health, and a number of dermatologic conditions can be traced to a specific vitamin deficiency or other nutritional deficit. But unlike, say, pellagra, which is caused by a lack of niacin and can be remedied by niacin supplements, there is no simple cause-and-effect or curative relationship between acne and any one nutritional element. Nonetheless, there are some key nutrients that some researchers feel seem to aid in the treatment of acne.

"I think it's a good idea to take vitamin supplements to make sure you're getting antioxidants, like vitamins A and C and E," says Cleveland dermatologist Wilma Bergfeld. "There isn't much research showing what they might do in acne, but there is enough interesting information out there about how antioxidants help your skin in general that I don't know of a single physician who isn't taking them—even if nothing has been proven."

Vitamin A

Vitamin A (retinol) is the source of the most potent of the proven prescription acne drugs—the topical retinoids such as Retin-A, and isotretinoin (Accutane). Adequate levels of vitamin A are important for maintaining skin health. It moderates cell turnover and sebum production, and in high doses has been shown to reduce both sebum and the buildup of keratinocytes in sebaceous follicles. Some dermatologists have successfully used ultra-high-dose vitamin A therapy—from 300,000 to 400,000 International Units (IU) per day for five to six months—to treat acne.

But these are astronomical, potentially toxic amounts that should never be taken except under a physician's care. Such high doses of vitamin A pose the risk of producing side effects similar to those of Accutane, including birth defects. In general, any amount over 10,000 IU per day, the FDA-established upper level for women, should be taken only under medical supervision. Women who are pregnant, or may become so, should not take more than the recommended daily allowance for pregnancy—2,565 IU.

"In my practice I use as a baseline a prescription multivitamin supplement with 8000 IU of A and 80 milligrams of zinc, both of which have been used independently to treat acne," says Bergfeld. "It's prescription because of the amounts of A and zinc. It keeps them higher than normal, but at a nontoxic level. And I think it helps get some really good results with acne patients."

Vitamin B Complex

The interrelated B vitamins are what are known as coenzymes, which means that they help enzymes carry out their functions in the body. They play an important role in energy production, nerve-signal transmission, and the synthesis of hormones. Although B vitamins should be taken together, several have been investigated separately as acne remedies.

Vitamin B_3 (niacin) has been used for years to treat inflammatory skin conditions, including acne, and an oral version is now available in a prescription acne medicine (page 134).

Vitamin B_5 (pantothenic acid) is important for fat metabolism and may have an effect on sebum production in the skin. In a Chinese study of one hundred subjects given both oral pantothenic acid and a topical cream containing the vitamin, the treatment appeared to both decrease sebum in the skin and reduce the number of inflammatory acne lesions.

Vitamin B_6 (pyridoxine) plays a role in the metabolism of steroid hormones. In experiments with rats, pyridoxine deficiency caused an increased sensitivity to testosterone, the hormone most involved in stimulating the sebaceous follicles. Pyridoxine is sometimes suggested as a supplement for women with premenstrual acne.

Dr. Jeanette Jacknin, an Arizona dermatologist who integrates alternative therapies into her practice, recommends in her book *Smart Medicine for Your Skin* a supplement that provides 100 milligrams of each of the major B vitamins daily for acne patients.

Vitamins C and E

Vitamins C and E are antioxidants that may play a role in muting the inflammation in acne. E, moreover, is essential for the proper functioning of vitamin A; if blood levels of E fall, vitamin A levels also decline. Jacknin suggests 400 IU of vitamin E daily, with 500 to 1,000 milligrams of vitamin C with bioflavonoids three times a day.

Selenium

The trace mineral selenium helps maximize the body's use of vitamin E, and aids in preventing inflammation. Some studies have shown that women with acne have less-than-normal amounts of selenium in their bodies. The recommended daily allowance of selenium is about 70 micrograms per day. Alternative healers suggest between 100 and 200 micrograms a day for acne, from food and supplement sources combined. Foods containing selenium include broccoli, brown rice, whole wheat, garlic, and tuna; one Brazil nut contains 120 micrograms. Caution: Selenium overdose (more than 400 micrograms a day over the long term) can produce toxic side effects such as fragile fingernails and hair loss.

Zinc

Zinc has a number of potential benefits for the skin. It is an essential mineral required for protein synthesis and collagen formation, it helps vitamin A function properly, and it is involved in testosterone regulation. It is also an anti-inflammatory agent, and may play a role in inhibiting the skin enzyme 5-alpha reductase, which converts testosterone into the sebum-stimulating hormone DHT. Oral zinc has never been conclusively shown to have a curative effect on acne, but some dermatologists suggest daily zinc supplements, containing anywhere from 25 to 100 milligrams, as an adjunctive treatment for inflammatory acne.

HERBAL TREATMENTS

Herbal medicines are prepared from a variety of botanical materials—leaves, stems, roots, berries, etc.—that contain biologically active ingredients. At least a quarter of all conventional prescription drugs include the same ingredients in purified form, and the use of herbal medicine is widely accepted in Europe. In fact, in Germany, doctors study herbal therapy in medical school, and a regulatory commission oversees herbal preparations. In the United States, on the other hand, herbal medicines are regarded as dietary supplements, and thus not regulated as drugs by the FDA. This means that they come in unpredictable strengths and the amounts of active ingredients vary greatly.

Prepared in various teas or infusions, or in the form of pills, capsules, and powders, the oral herbal medicines commonly recommended for acne come from across the spectrum of alternative medicine, with different traditions recommending different herbs for the same problem.

"There are things in some of those herbal remedies, some of those Chinese herbs, that may have some positive merit for treating acne. Some of them, for example, have anti-androgen activity," explains Bergfeld. "But you have to be careful, because with so little standardization, the levels of purity are somewhat questionable. Say there's a tree that has a berry or a flower that might be therapeutic. But it grows somewhere like Afghanistan. You don't know if that plant is healthy. You don't know if it has been sprayed with pesticides or other chemicals. You don't know what kind of climate problems it has. Then they mix it in with a bunch of other stuff, and you just have no idea what's in it. You can't just go and use these things if you don't know where they're from and what's in them. It's too much of a risk."

Aside from questions of purity, herbal medicines can be quite potent and may have unpredictable side effects. You would be well advised to take them only under the guidance of a health-care practitioner who is familiar with their properties.

Saw Palmetto

Saw palmetto is a tropical berry that acts as an anti-androgen. It is often recommended to men as an herbal supplement to promote prostate gland health. When taken orally, saw palmetto reduces the body's production of 5-alpha reductase, the skin enzyme that converts testosterone into sebum-stimulating DHT.

Vitex

Vitex is a fruit extract listed as an acne treatment by the German Regulatory Commission E (the official body that controls herbal medicine in Germany). Taken orally, Vitex has been shown to be effective in treating premenstrual acne. It is believed to work by regulating the two pituitary hormones— follicle stimulating hormone (FSH) and luteinizing hormone (LH)—that stimulate the ovaries. It should not be taken by pregnant or nursing women.

TOPICAL TREATMENTS

Dozens of topically applied herbal-, mineral-, or animal-derived alternative ingredients now show up in the brand-name acne products of major cosmetic and pharmaceutical companies, as well as mixed into products of doctors who market their own skin-care lines. Dr. Perricone, for example, has developed a small group of acne products that contain many of the same antioxidant and anti-inflammatory agents that he recommends for the treatment of aging skin: DMAE, tyrosine, alpha lipoic acid, green tea extract, allantoin, soy, chamomile, glutathione.

None of these ingredients, or the many others you can find in the acne medicines from companies such as Estée Lauder (parent company of Clinique), Johnson & Johnson (Neutrogena, Clean & Clear, and Aveeno), and Proctor & Gamble (Olay and Bioré) have been extensively researched as dermatological agents, much less as acne drugs. Like herbal medicines taken by mouth, they are not regulated as drugs in the United States, and so their precise therapeutic qualities are essentially an open question.

However, many of them are generally recognized to have anti-inflammatory or anti-irritant qualities that make them theoretically helpful for treating inflammatory acne lesions. Others, when tested in small trials, have shown other qualities that make them at least plausible as topical acne fighters.

Anti-inflammatory Botanicals

For the most part, the host of botanical ingredients incorporated into acne products are put there for their anti-inflammatory, anti-irritant, or antioxidant properties. Glutathione, goldenseal, grape root, DMAE, lipoic acid, tyrosine, allantoin, sucrose, and kola nut, to name just a few, all have qualities that can help calm red acne lesions, even though, overwhelmingly, most of the tests that have been done on them have investigated their prowess in fighting other inflammatory conditions. In experiments with albino rats, for example, the freeze-dried extract of calendula (pot marigold), commonly recommended as an acne fighter, was shown to suppress inflammation and infiltration of leukocytes (white blood cells). German chamomile has a centuries-old tradition as a skin treatment; its main constituent, a chemical called alpha bisabolol, helps wounds to heal and is an anti-inflammatory agent. The dried flower heads of arnica (*Arnica montana L.*), in the form of a tincture, are reputed to prevent and reduce inflammation and provide some antibiotic properties against acne lesions.

Green Tea Extract

Consumed around the world as a beverage, green tea is also a popular ingredient in many cosmetic products. Several studies investigating its effects on sun-damaged skin have shown that topically applied green tea extracts have both anti-inflammatory and antioxidant activity that counters the destructive impact of ultraviolet light. Green tea extracts may also work to inhibit the enzyme 5-alpha reductase (which converts testosterone into the sebaceous gland–stimulating hormone, DHT), and thus conceivably could help reduce sebum production in acne patients. A small 2001 university study on the effects of green tea on acne compared a cream containing 2 percent green tea extract with a placebo cream on sixty patients with moderate acne. At the end of sixteen weeks, the patients who had been using the cream with green tea had seen about a 75 percent clearance of their lesions, versus the placebo group, which had experienced only about a 7 percent improvement.

Isolutrol

"Isolutrol" is a name given to a substance extracted from the gallbladder or liver of sharks. It is found in a skin-care line called Ketsugo. At least one Japanese study suggested that topically applied isolutrol may inhibit sebum production. A 1995 clinical trial on seventy patients with mild to moderate acne compared a preparation containing isolutrol with a 5 percent benzoyl peroxide lotion (which inhibits bacteria). It found that both treatments reduced inflamed lesions, although isolutrol, unlike benzoyl peroxide, did not also significantly reduce the number of blackheads and whiteheads. The patients treated with isolutrol experienced fewer side effects than those treated with benzoyl peroxide.

Niacinamide

Topical niacinamide, the active form of vitamin B_3, is a cosmeceutical ingredient with a broad range of potential benefits for improving the appearance of photo-damaged skin. It represses the transfer of melanin from the pigment-producing melanocytes to cells on the skin surface, which helps improve the appearance of hyperpigmented spots. Several small studies have indicated that a topical 4 percent niacinamide gel is effective in reducing acne papules and pustules. It is available commercially in a product called Papulex and also as a component in VitaNiacin, a trademarked combination of vitamin E, panthenol (a form of vitamin B_5), and niacinamide found in the Oil of Olay Total Effects line of antiaging products from Procter & Gamble.

Soy

Widely recognized for a variety of health benefits when eaten as food, soy contains a number of components that may also eventually prove to make it useful in topical skin care products. Those potentially beneficial in treating acne include unsaturated fatty acids that may provide antioxidant effects, and surfactants that might provide cleaning activity; soy phytoestrogens (plant compounds that have an estrogen-like effect) could have an effect on skin similar to that of topical estrogen, working to increase skin thickness and help block the androgens that contribute to acne. Moreover, soy proteins appear to inhibit skin pigmentation, making them a possible supplementary treatment for pigmentation disorders—including the hyperpigmented macules that arise on dark skin in the wake of acne lesions.

In a small clinical trial conducted by Johnson & Johnson, twenty-six women with mild acne were given a moisturizer containing a soy formulation to apply twice a day for thirty-five days. Both pimples and skin redness diminished in four weeks. Johnson & Johnson's Aveeno skin-care products contain the soy formula.

Tea Tree Oil

In recent years, tea tree oil has become increasingly popular as an alternative to conventional over-the-counter acne medicines. Several manufacturers have incorporated it as an ingredient in their products, and the pure oil is widely available in health food stores.

Tea tree oil comes from the leaves of a small tree (called Melaleuca), native to only one region of the world: the northeast coastal region of New South Wales, Australia. It is a traditional antiseptic and antifungal skin disinfectant, used by aboriginal Australians for centuries. Early European settlers used it as an antiseptic for cuts, abrasions, burns, and athlete's foot. Tea tree oil penetrates the skin well, and has been shown in laboratory tests to be effective against a wide range of organisms, including *P. acnes*.

Tea tree oil's reputation as an acne fighter rests largely on a study done in 1990, at the Royal Prince Hospital in New South Wales. The results showed that a solution containing 5 percent tea tree oil was as effective at reducing inflamed acne lesions as a solution containing 5 percent benzoyl peroxide. The tea tree oil did not work as quickly as the benzoyl peroxide, but it produced fewer side effects. (Tea tree oil is generally regarded as safe for most patients; in some users, however, it may cause mild contact dermatitis or eczema.)

Because tea tree oil is not regulated as a drug by the FDA, manufacturers who include it in anti-acne treatments do not have to disclose the percentage they are using (although some companies do, in fact, put that information on the label). However, a look at various ingredient labels (which list ingredients in descending order) suggests that tea tree oil is typically present in far less than the 5 percent range. For example, Burt's Bees Herbal Blemish Stick lists tea tree oil as an ingredient in tenth place, which typically would put it in the 1-percent-or-less range. An alternative is the pure essential oil; however, it is more likely to produce side effects such as contact dermatitis.

Topical Zinc

In laboratory tests, zinc is a potent inhibitor of neutrophils, the white blood cells that play such a significant role in inflammatory acne. Zinc is valued as an exceptionally safe topical anti-inflammatory agent in medicines for other skin conditions. (For example, it is the principal ingredient in many diaper rash ointments.) But tests of its prowess as an acne fighter have been mixed. In trials conducted many years ago, a topical formulation of zinc plus erythromycin showed itself to be more effective against acne than erythromycin alone. (The combination is marketed overseas as the acne medicine Zineryt.) Subsequent trials have failed to demonstrate impressive effects on acne, although zinc is incorporated into a number of over-the-counter acne preparations, as well as in the prescription benzoyl peroxide line Triaz.

TRADITIONAL CHINESE MEDICINE

Traditional Chinese Medicine (TCM) is a centuries-old holistic system of health care that incorporates the use of medicinal herbs, acupuncture, nutritional therapy, massage, and exercise. It is estimated that one quarter of the world's population employs at least some form of TCM therapy, and it has been shown to be effective for many conditions, including acne.

It is difficult to directly compare TCM's approach to healing, which looks for underlying imbalances and disharmonies in the body and seeks to correct them, with Western medical practice. But researchers have speculated that in treating skin disease, many elements of Chinese medicine work synergistically to address various aspects of the inflammatory process. Moreover, two studies investigating the effects of acupuncture on women with acne concluded that the technique influenced the hormonal mechanisms that trigger breakouts. In one of the studies, electromagnetic acupuncture treatment regulated the hormonal irregularities of women with polycystic ovaries and alleviated their acne.

HOMEOPATHY

Homeopathy, a holistic health-care system founded in the late 1800s by a German physician named Samuel Hahnemann, is based on the principle that "like cures like." Hahnemann believed that if a large dose of something could cause a healthy person to contract a given disease or set of symptoms, then an infinitesimal dose of the same thing would activate a sick body into fighting off that disease or those same symptoms. This is somewhat similar to the principle behind allergy shots, in which a small dose of an allergen is given to a person in order to stimulate the body's ability to fend off a more potent assault by a substance that would provoke an allergic reaction.

Homeopathic remedies are created through a process of successively diluting therapeutic substances in pure water or alcohol. Remedies are made into liquids or tablets, which are regulated by the FDA as over-the-counter medicines. The various formulas, created through years of trial-and-error experimentation, are arcanely expressed in enigmatic ratios meant to reflect the degree of dilution. For instance, the strength designated as "1x" indicates a mixture of one part substance to nine parts dilution medium.

Homeopathy is practiced throughout the world, but there is scant scientific evidence to back up its claims, and there have been no well-designed studies examining its use in acne. In Britain, homeopathic hospital and outpatient clinics are included in the national health-care system. "But I have not seen it to be very effective against acne," comments Dr. Anthony Chu, a British dermatologist and founder of the British Acne Support Group.

There are a number of system-specific homeopathic remedies for acne. A combination of the most frequently used remedies can be found over the counter in a two-part acne treatment product called Nature's Cure. The package contains homeopathic acne tablets made in accordance with the Homeopathic Pharmacopoeia of the United States, and a nicely formulated 5 percent benzoyl peroxide vanishing cream—a complementary acne treatment package all in one.

Chapter Ten

The Mind-Skin Connection

DERMATOLOGISTS SAY THAT MORE WOMEN acne patients attribute their breakouts to stress than to any other single cause. And certainly most acne-prone women have plenty of anecdotal experience to back those perceptions up.

"You've got a presentation to give at work, your little girl gets a cold, and you have to stay home for six hours until the sitter gets there," says Chicago's Dr. Marianne O'Donoghue, outlining a familiar scenario. "You're trying to appease your boss, take care of your child, straighten up your house, and, at the same time, finish your project. If you have acne-prone skin, you just know you're going to have three new pimples in a heartbeat."

But while the cause-and-effect connection between having acne and having a bad day is as obvious to acne-plagued modern women as the proverbial elephant in the middle of the room, there has been, until recently, surprisingly little research to either explain it or back it up.

"Nobody has *ever* demonstrated convincingly that stress induces acne," asserts Munich's Professor Gerd Plewig. "Everybody writes about it. Patients claim it; doctors confirm it; but I have not seen any serious effort to prove it. I'm not saying that stress hormones don't have an effect on your acne, but, I repeat, nobody has ever really proven it."

Other doctors concede that may be true, but believe that stress is nonetheless a major element of many a modern woman's acne outbreaks—just as it is widely recognized to be a potent aggravating factor in other common inflammatory skin conditions, such as psoriasis and eczema. "The old days, when we sat back and said nothing when acne patients talked about stress, are over," says dermatologist and clinical psychologist Richard Fried, of Yardley, Pennsylvania, a specialist in the growing field of psychodermatology, the science of skin and emotions. "Physicians used to either dismiss the connection or tacitly validate it, but never really take the next step and say, 'What is the actual mechanism at work here?' Well, we now know enough about the mechanisms of stress to see that the role it plays in acne is not a mysterious black box."

NOWHERE TO RUN

The connection between acne and stress does, in fact, apparently lie in the effects of stress on the complex workings of the endocrine system. When your body is subjected to either emotional or physical stress (the latter can be caused by fatigue, lack of sleep, crash dieting, and drinking or smoking, among other stressors), it reacts in much the same way its primitive ancestral forebears did when encountering a predator or foe. The adrenal glands go into overdrive, pouring out the so-called "fight-or-flight" stress hormones, cortisol and epinephrine (also called adrenaline), which prepare you to flee from the prowling beast or fight your enemy.

But in the modern world, there is usually nowhere to run and few acceptable ways to battle a perceived enemy, whether it's a tyrannical boss or a careening road hog. So the hormones build up, and may act on your skin in two ways to give you acne.

One is a long-term effect, due to the fact that along with those fight-or-flight hormones come other adrenal hormones, including the androgens that stimulate sebaceous glands and promote the other cellular changes that create acne-inciting microcomedones in the sebaceous follicles. Thus, chronic, long-term stress may work to worsen existing acne, create new pimples in previously clear skin, and make your face feel oilier than normal.

The short-term effect—angry, red blemishes that seem to blossom before your very eyes—is apparently due to the heightened levels of cortisol (which provokes irritation, inflammation, and itchiness in the skin) and other inflammatory chemicals that flood the body in response to stressful situations. These substances can both aggravate existing blemishes and incite an intense inflammatory reaction in follicles that contain previously undetected microcomedones, quickly transforming them into those big acne pimples that erupt overnight.

Of course, these hormonal mechanisms do not cause acne in everyone. But just as some people are prone to digestive disorders or migraines when under stress, others appear programmed to break out. "If a woman has normal skin, having a bad day is probably not going to give her acne, " emphasizes O'Donoghue. "But if she has acne-prone skin, she's going to get zits when she is stressed or worn out. She's got the fertile soil, which is the acne-prone skin. And she's got the seeds— the microcomedones. Then stress stimulates the adrenals, and everything just blows up."

THE VICIOUS CYCLE: ACNE PROVOKING ACNE

For many women with acne, the skin-stress connection is cruelly exacerbated by yet another insidious connection—the fact that acne itself is stressful. Not only does it toy with your emotions by making you feel self-conscious and eroding your self-esteem, but it also keeps you hanging in the unnerving state of never knowing what will happen next. Fried says that the results are similar to those attained in a classic laboratory experiment involving rats.

A researcher takes a rat and puts it in a cage equipped with two levers. When the rat presses one lever, he gets an electric shock; when he presses the other, he gets food. In fairly short order, the rat learns to avoid the lever that shocks him and head for the one that gives him food when he is hungry. "And he's a happy, emotionally well-adjusted rat," says Fried. "His life is predictable, and he feels in control of his environment. He eats normally, he's got a healthy immune system. If you put other rats in the cage with him, he will socialize appropriately with them; he will mate normally with a female rat."

If, on the other hand, the scientist puts a rat in a cage with two identical levers, but continuously switches the wiring around so that the rat never knows which one will shock him and which one will reward him with food, he soon becomes a basket case. "These rats become hostile or withdrawn; they overeat or refuse to eat; their immune systems go haywire, and they come down with diseases; they become sexually apathetic or hypersexual; sometimes they engage in autistic rocking behavior."

The difference is that the second rat is living in a completely unpredictable environment with no sense of control over what happens to him. You can apply that model, says Fried, to human beings living in any unpredictable environment—whether it's a war zone or a household with an alcoholic. They get stressed; they feel anxious; they may get eating disorders, become promiscuous or sexually inactive; they feel anger; they feel depression.

"Well, what is acne, after all," asks Fried, "but totally unpredictable? Its absolutely capricious nature is one of its worst characteristics. The acne patient lives with the sense she can never be completely sure about what will happen next, that she has no control over her own skin. She's using her Benza-Clin, she's using her Tazorac, and then suddenly her acne is worse than it was two weeks ago. Of course it's stressful. How could it not be?"

TAKING CONTROL

Whatever science ultimately proves or disproves about the precise mechanisms that connect acne with emotions, if stress makes your acne worse, you are probably already well aware of it. And anything you can do to relieve tension or anxiety stands to benefit both your general health and your complexion.

Essentially, the goal is to condition your immune system so that it behaves in a more modulated and appropriate fashion to stressful situations. Specifically, so that it does not react to stress by flooding your body with chemicals that kindle the kind of out-of-control inflammation that is so apt to ignite your acne.

According to Fried, employing strategies that enhance a sense of control is pivotal. "Study after study shows that the more in control people feel, the less stress they feel and the fewer negative sensations they experience."

Some established methods for reducing stress and gaining that sense of control include the following:

1. Exercise. Engage in some form of regular physical activity, within your own capacity and interests, even if is just a brief daily walk. After all, a stressed-out body is one that is chemically primed to fight or flee; mov-

ing is what it needs to do. "I think exercise is key," emphasizes Fried. "Study after study is has shown that exercise reduces stress. And that people who exercise tend to feel more in control of their lives."

2. Formal stress reduction techniques. Meditation, prayer, tai chi, yoga, progressive muscle relaxation, among many other such methods, similarly act to modulate the production of stress hormones and enhance a sense of control.

3. Proactive skin care. If you happen to be having one of those days when your child is sick, the boss is clamoring, the sitter is a no-show, etc., you may not have time to fit in a visit to the yoga studio or go for a run. But what you can do, presuming you are already on a regular acne-preventive skin-care regimen, is make doubly sure that you don't neglect it. In fact, you might actually want to step it up a bit. For example, if you've been using a topical, over-the-counter medicine once a day, you may want to apply it two or three times a day for a week or so (until your life calms down), or you may want to use a slightly higher potency. Or, if you're seeing a dermatologist, ask if there are any ways you can adjust your prescription medication during stressful periods, just as dermatologists sometimes prescribe intensified treatment (higher dosages or additional medicines) to head off premenstrual flares. "I also encourage acne patients to take full advantage of spot treatments and camouflage makeup," adds Fried. "It's another way of helping them feel more in control."

4. Face down feelings of guilt or failure. The complex feelings of shame and responsibility that afflict many acne

patients can exacerbate stress and sabotage other stress-management techniques. Talk to a physician. Read up; learn everything you can. The more you know about acne, the more you will be able to recognize and accept that it really is not your fault.

Says Fried: "If I could address an open letter to all acne patients, I'd say this: 'It happened strictly because in your genes there was a tendency for your follicles to misbehave. And it was just a matter of time—whether it was puberty, or turning thirty-two, or losing your job—before this unfolded. It was nothing you did, and you couldn't have stopped it.' "

5. Seek professional assistance. If you feel you need extra help, psychotherapists have additional stress-alleviating tools: traditional talk therapy to help you gain perspective and insight, mind-body training techniques such as hypnosis or biofeedback, and prescription medicines. Many of the same drugs that are widely used to treat depression and anxiety are now also believed to directly affect the way skin responds to inflammatory stimuli.

BUT WILL ALL THIS CURE YOUR ACNE?

Stress reduction is probably not in and of itself a "cure" for anyone's acne. But it certainly can play a role in managing acne-prone skin, according to Fried, who says he tells his acne patients this:

"I unquestionably believe that stress can make the skin more reactive, and that can worsen acne. Conversely, the more we can do to control your stress, the better your skin will do.

Purely from a physiological point of view, managing stress better and stopping those massive cortisol outpourings has got to create a friendlier environment for those follicles. However, that does not mean that if tonight you have a nasty breakout, you screwed up and inadequately handled your stress. It's much like the meditation and relaxation techniques many cancer patients now use. We know those patients do better, we know they live longer, but does it mean that if they have a recurrence, it's their fault? Of course not.

"By the same token, you can't look at any given pimple on any given day or week and say that it is a measure of your success or failure. We are talking about learning skills that overall will help your body to be healthier and function better. So, I say to every one of my acne patients who is doing something proactively to manage stress, 'You know what? I will guarantee you, if you weren't doing what you are doing, you would have more acne and you would be using more medicine. So this is by no means a wasted effort.'"

Chapter Eleven

⸺◦⸺

Looking Good

THERE IS NO GETTING AROUND THE FACT that effective acne treatment really is all about prevention. It's an endless, on-going coaxing of the skin into behaving normally so that it won't produce any new breakouts. But even as you are working to get your acne under control, what do you do about the blemishes that are already there? What if a new one pops up despite all your care? And what about oil slicks and makeup that seems to slide off your shiny skin? How can you manage to look good when your skin still looks so bad?

SPOT TREATMENT

For starters, you can always do what acne-plagued models and actresses do before they hit the catwalk or the red carpet with no airbrushing or digital tricks to conceal their breakouts: rush to a dermatologist at the first sign of trouble. A professional shot of a corticosteroid injected directly into an inflamed zit will stop the inflammation in its tracks and shrink the pimple into obscurity within hours.

This is strong medicine—definitely not something you can do every day, or for every pimple on your face if you've got active acne. (Repeated injections of corticosteroids can cause skin to atrophy.) But it really is the most effective thing you can do in an acne emergency—the secret weapon of high-profile public women (and savvy brides) who count on having flawless-appearing complexions for their photo shoots, their public appearances, and their wedding days.

Of course, you do need to already be seeing a dermatologist; you're not likely to find a doctor who'll inject your zits for you on an emergency basis if you're not already a regular patient. And you won't be able to do it every week. But it's good to know that there is a way to get rid of a big breakout fast if you really have to.

If you're on your own, there are a few other things you can do to minimize a pimple or slow its progress. At the very first sign that trouble is brewing—when you sense the first little bit of heat, soreness, or pressure deep down in your skin—apply ice. Take an ice cube and hold it or rub it over the spot for a couple of minutes, two or three times a day. This is not the time for soothing warm compresses. "Definitely ice rather than heat at this stage," says Chicago dermatologist Marianne O' Donoghue. "It slows the inflammation. If you are getting an inflamed pimple and you give it heat, it will bring in more blood and it's going to be a big pimple—a big, humongous pimple."

Acne expert Dr. James Fulton, one the developers of Retin-A, is another firm believer in ice treatment. He writes in his book, *Acne RX*, that icing a pimple not only helps to reduce the swelling and redness, but makes the outer surface of the skin somewhat more permeable to topical medicines. In fact, Fulton recommends that all acne patients apply ice to affected areas of skin twice a day, before applying any medicine. So, after using the ice, apply a topical antibiotic medicine if you have one (it will both reduce the inflammation itself and attack the *P. acnes* bacteria inciting it) or benzoyl peroxide.

Sometimes the ice and the antibacterial medicine does the trick, and the incipient zit dies down. If it does not, and instead grows into a raised pimple, it's time to try one of the commercial spot treatments containing an anti-inflammatory agent, such as sulfur, sulfur and resorcinol, or salicylic acid. "About twenty-eight years ago we did tests showing that a lot of these products, like salicylic acid and sulfur and resorcinol—the old products—really can help accelerate the resolution of a pimple," says SUNY's Alan Shalita. "Let's say that if it takes an average pimple or papule ten to twelve days to go away by itself, maybe this will reduce it to eight or nine days. It won't cut the time in half, but it inhibits the neutrophils, it takes a little of the water out, it kind of dries things up. So it helps."

Once you have a fully developed pimple, benzoyl peroxide, which acts primarily on live bacteria, becomes relatively less effective. At this point, you're fighting full-blown inflammation, and the bacteria that played such a key role in setting it off have by now been decimated by neutrophils and other inflammatory chemicals. But ice continues to help at this stage, so keep using it. "You can also speed things up with a topical antibiotic," adds Shalita. "Or adapalene [Differin], which has also been shown to have anti-inflammatory properties."

You can also try to alleviate inflammation with an over-the-counter nonsteroidal anti-inflammatory pain medication such as ibuprofen (Advil). Shalita is skeptical ("I think that to see any real effect, you would need to take more than is really prudent"), but one eight-week study, reported on at a 2002 dermatology meeting in Brazil, found that acne patients who took 1,200 milligrams of ibuprofen each day, along with their 150-milligram daily dose of the prescription antibiotic minocycline, saw more improvement in their inflamed acne lesions than did patients who took only the minocycline.

(Package directions for adults taking Advil for pain recommend a 200-milligram tablet every four to eight hours, not to
exceed six pills in twenty-four hours.)

One other possibility—and again you will need a dermatologist for this—is a strong topical prescription cortisone medication. "I don't recommend it, except in very rare cases," says
Shalita. "But you can take a very high concentration of hydrocortisone derivatives and just apply it to the spot, like when
we inject them. You run the risk of getting chronically dilated
blood vessels in that spot, so I only will give this to patients
who I'm really comfortable with and who I can instruct
exactly how to do it. And that I know I can trust to not overuse it." Don't expect mild, over-the-counter hydrocortisone
creams, like Cortaid, to have much impact on blemishes.
"They're not strong enough to make a difference," says Shalita.

POPPING PIMPLES?

Do not *ever* try to pop, squeeze, or otherwise manipulate an
inflamed pimple that is just a red, headless bump, deep in your
skin. There is no way you can get it out, "bring it to a head," or
do anything else but make the inflammation worse, longer
lasting, and much more likely to leave a permanent scar.

The rule about action becomes more equivocal, though,
once a lesion has turned into an obvious pustule with a yellow
or whitish head. The white dot is a sign of pus coming to the
surface, possibly carrying with it the little comedo that started
the problem in the first place. This is the point when, really,
you cannot stand the way it looks, and you're dying to do
something. And just about every piece of sensible advice
you've ever heard tells you not to touch it! That is definitely
the prudent course: Just keep applying the ice and the spot

treatment and wait for the pimple to resolve on its own. Eventually it will open up, drain, and heal.

But if you are daring, defiant even, and insist on doing something, you could try the following. First, carefully clean your skin and apply a warm moist compress for a few minutes. Next, take a fine sewing needle, sterilize it in alcohol (don't use a match flame; it will deposit carbon on the needle, and you could wind up tattooing yourself), and use it to puncture the skin over the yellow head. Then just let the lesion drain and blot it with a tissue. If you can't help yourself, very gently and lightly press (with clean, tissue-padded fingers) down around the edges of the lesion. Stop immediately and apply ice if you see blood or clear liquid serum; these are signs that you are damaging the skin and making the pimple worse.

In *Acne RX*, Dr. Fulton describes a more aggressive approach aimed at extracting the comedo so that it won't get left behind to seed a new pimple. It requires a steady hand and a lot of nerve. Look carefully at the lesion (a magnifying mirror helps a lot here) to find the tiny central pore and determine its slant; you may be able to figure this out by the direction in which little facial hairs in the area grow. Then insert the sterilized needle, at that angle, about one-sixteenth of an inch into the opening of the pore. If you do not get any blood or serum (signs you've missed the natural opening, and that you should stop and apply ice), move the needle just a tiny bit from side to side to slightly widen the opening. Then, using your padded fingers, gently press down and in, around the pimple. You are trying to expel just white pus and a minute mass of hard material (the comedo).

If that doesn't happen, Fulton suggests waiting five to ten minutes and trying gentle pressure just one more time. If *that* doesn't work, stop. The more you monkey around with it, the worse the lesion will look, the longer it will take to heal, and the more likely it will be to leave a visible scar.

EXTRACTING BLACKHEADS AND WHITEHEADS

Compared to the hazards of dealing with an inflamed acne lesion, extracting open or closed comedones (blackheads and whiteheads) seems a relatively simple and straightforward undertaking. Comedo extractors—metal instruments that allow you to eject a comedo from its follicle by applying even pressure around its circumference—are widely available and easy to use. You can also use "pore strips"—pieces of cloth impregnated with a glue-like substance. Press one of these onto your nose. When you then pull the pore strip off, it may lift away the top layer of the epidermis and the plugs in the pores beneath. Pore strips have become a standard offering of many skin-care lines.

But comedo extraction, by any method, has a surprising number of pitfalls.

Doctors Plewig and Kligman's always illuminating textbook, *Acne and Rosacea*, devotes a full fourteen pages to the subject, with huge photographs of biopsied skin specimens to illustrate the ruinous consequences of poor or careless technique: inflammation, swelling, tiny ruptured blood vessels, little abscesses and other pockets of infection, tattered follicular walls. Even the most meticulous procedure typically leaves surprising amounts of material behind to start up a new comedo. And even if you succeed in completely emptying the follicle, unless you have also removed its encapsulating epithelial lining (a little sack of thin skin), Plewig and Kligman warn that it will immediately resume "its career of comedo-building."

You will know if you have been successful in extricating the epithelial lining, by the way, if the comedo comes out trailing a filmy tail. But that rarely happens without applying a lot of pressure and inflicting at least some damage to surrounding tissues. Removing closed comedones is even trickier, because the constricted pore must first be carefully dilated with a fine scalpel blade or other sharp instrument before you can press out the whitehead.

It is little wonder that most dermatologists advise patients not to try this at home, but to put their faces in the hands of a trained doctor, nurse, or aesthetician. It is good advice. Some dermatology offices do "acne surgery," as comedo removal is called, as a part of acne therapy. "I've been doing this on patients every day for more than twenty-five years!" says Atlanta's Dr. Harold Brody, one the nation's most esteemed dermatologic surgeons, of the humble chore.

Others, on the other hand, think the whole exercise is kind of pointless. "Why?" demanded Fairfax, Virginia, dermatologist Robert Silverman, when I inquired if his office performed comedo extractions. "Just use a topical retinoid; the blackheads should all be gone in three or four months."

In fact, getting and staying on a regimen of topical retinoids *is* the best way to get rid of comedones and keep clear of them. However, while you are waiting for a retinoid to do its leisurely work, ridding yourself of large obvious blackheads can yield a quick and satisfying improvement in your appearance.

If you insist on trying to do this yourself, wait until you've been on a retinoid or a salicylic acid product on the area for three or four weeks; the blackheads will come out much more easily and you will do less damage. Then, get a good comedo extractor. (The worst damage comes from using your fingers; even if you think you've been gentle, and don't see any damage, pressing with your fingers creates havoc below the surface.) Try to find an extractor with a generously sized opening; the tiny holes on some drugstore brands squeeze too tightly around the follicle. One of the best is called the Schaumberg Extractor, which is available through medical and beauty supply houses (your pharmacist can order it for you); it has a longish, oval-shaped opening which can fit around any blackhead.

Pore strips are out, by the way, if you are using a topical retinoid or any of the cosmetic exfoliants such as salicylic or glycolic acid; they make the skin too vulnerable to injury. If you are not on a retinoid, and *do* want to try pore strips, Dr. Susan Bershad cautions that you should use them only on your nose. "On other parts of your face they pull out these little peach-fuzz hairs; when they start to grow back, they can get caught under the skin and create little pustules."

By all means, avoid any of the battery-powered vacuum cleaner–like pore-suction devices. They're not effective and they can injure the skin; they will give you what look like little hickeys. I once came across a note on an acne treatment products website that kind of said it all: "We no longer offer the electric suction–type pore cleaners because of the return rate and they just don't work as well as the reliable extractors do."

OIL BLOTTERS

The oldest and most common method of dealing with facial oiliness is to swab the skin down with an alcohol-based astringent or toner. These instantly dissolve and remove surface oil, and can be handy in a pinch. But they do nothing to minimize the presence of oil throughout the day. And they can be irritating to boot.

For more lasting shine control, there are cosmetic products containing sebum-absorbing minerals such as magnesium aluminum silicate or magnesium hydroxide. Depending on how naturally oily your skin is to begin with, their effects can last from a couple of hours to half a day.

Milk of magnesia, which is the liquid form of magnesium hydroxide, both soaks up oil and helps to soothe the skin. Cosmetic consumer writer Paula Begoun, author of *The Beauty Bible* and *Don't Go to the Cosmetics Counter Without Me*, swears by plain unflavored milk of magnesia from the drugstore as one of the best and least-expensive oil absorbers around, and she sells a cosmetic version as part of her Paula's Choice skin-care line. Begoun recommends applying a thin layer of milk of magnesia under makeup as a kind of spackle, to help fill in visible pores and provide an even base for foundation. This also helps keep your foundation from migrating, which is a particularly evident problem with oily skin.

Facial treatments containing specialized oil-absorbing chemicals have a much longer-lasting effect. A product called Seban soaks up sebum with a chemical called a "perfluoroalkyl surfactant," porous chemical particles, or "micro-sponges"— somewhat like the chemical package that contains the active ingredient tretinoin in Retin-A Micro. Seban is formulated in an alcohol-based liquid; its manufacturer claims it should keep you looking oil-free for about eight hours.

Clinac OC Oil Control Gel contains a patented polymer molecule, based on technology originally developed to clean up oil spills in the ocean, that absorbs oil and breaks it down into harmless substances. In a 2003 article in *Skin and Allergy News*, Dr. Leslie Baumann, director of cosmetic dermatology at the University of Miami, suggests mixing Clinac Gel with sunscreen, which gives you oil control and sun protection in one application, and reduces the greasy appearance that some sunscreens impart. She writes that studies have shown that combining the two does not impair the effectiveness of the sunscreen.

Both Seban and Clinac OC are nonprescription products, but they may not be readily available in retail outlets. (See appendix for mail-order sources.)

MOISTURIZERS AND SUNSCREENS

Many women with acne do not need a moisturizer—or, heaven forbid, a night cream or a nourishing cream or any other kind of rich emollient skin treatment. "American women are so *brainwashed* about moisturizers," exclaims New York dermatologist Laurie Polis. "Moisturizers are fine if you have dry skin, but if you don't, what are you doing? Giving yourself more acne, that's what!"

However, if you have superficial dry or flaking areas—which is a very likely prospect if you are starting up with a new topical acne medicine—an oil-free, non-comedogenic moisturizer can help to counteract the peeling. Use it judiciously, just on the areas where it is needed.

During the day, your sunscreen can serve as a moisturizer. And you should be wearing a sunscreen. The American Academy of Dermatology (AAD) recommends that everyone apply a sunscreen with an SPF of at least 15 every day to protect skin against carcinogenic ultraviolet light. Sunscreen is particularly crucial for acne patients because most acne treatments make your skin even more sensitive to the sun.

Sunscreen is doubly critical for dark-skinned acne patients, who may not customarily wear sun-protection products, relying instead on their natural pigment to protect them from ultraviolet damage. But even the smallest amount of sunlight (including sunlight through a window) exacerbates post-inflammatory hyperpigmentation. It will not only make dark, hyperpigmented acne macules even darker, but it will also sabotage the effects of any skin-lightening medicines you may be using to diminish the spots.

Sunscreens often cause breakouts in people with acne-prone or sensitive skin. Dr. Zoe Diana Draelos, clinical associate professor of dermatology at Wake Forest University and an expert on facial cosmetics, has hypothesized that the culprits are not the usual suspects—typical comedogenic or acnegenic agents—but the chemical sunscreening agents themselves. The chemical sunscreens (common examples include oxybenzone and avobenzone) that are found in the vast majority of sun protection products work by absorbing ultraviolet light. This creates heat energy—which is why sunscreens make some people feel hot. In susceptible skin, the heat, in turn, can cause acneiform eruptions—small papules and pustules—twenty-four to forty-eight hours later. So sunscreens containing only the physical sun-blocking agents titanium dioxide or zinc oxide are generally the best choice for people who find that sunscreens make them break out.

FACIAL FOUNDATIONS

For women with acne, foundation makeup can be either a trusted friend that shields your blemishes from the world, or a heartless foe that cruelly calls attention to them—often adding injury to insult by making the breakouts worse. It all depends on what you choose and how you use it.

Choosing a foundation can be confusing because cosmetic companies today make so many varieties for every conceivable skin type. But they can all be sorted into one of four basic categories: oil-based, water-free, water-based, and oil-free.

Oil-based foundations are water-in-oil emulsions, in which particles of colored pigment are suspended in an oil, such as mineral oil, lanolin, or vegetable oil; the pigment-containing oil is then mixed with water. When the makeup is applied, the water evaporates, leaving a smooth coating of the pigment-saturated oil on the skin. These makeups are a boon to dry-skinned women who need help keeping moisture in their skin.

In water-free (sometimes called "anhydrous") foundations, the oil-containing pigment is incorporated into waxes, which makes a thick, highly opaque substance that comes in a tube, a stick, or packed into a jar or tin. Water-free makeup is typically used as stage makeup or to camouflage facial scarring, bruising, or birthmarks.

Water-based foundations are oil-in-water emulsions, containing the same types of oils that are found in the oil-based products, but in smaller quantities. These usually come in a bottle and are most appropriate for normal or slightly dry skin. Although the term *water-based* may lead you to think these are suitable for oily or acne-prone skin, they are not. Even the relatively small amounts of oil they contain may contribute to breakouts and will certainly add additional shine to an already oily surface—highlighting textural anomalies such as pimples, scars, or large pores.

The fourth type of makeup, oil-free foundations, are best for oily and acne-prone complexions. These contain no animal, vegetable, or mineral oils. Instead, the pigments are typically incorporated into silicones, such as dimethicone or cyclomethicone, which are non-comedogenic, non-acnegenic, and hypoallergenic. They leave the skin, at least initially, with a slightly dry feeling, and they yield a matte or semimatte surface that helps to minimize surface irregularities.

Try not to confuse "oil-control" and "oil-free." All foundations, even oil-based ones, contain a certain amount of covering and "blotting" material (e.g., talc, starch, or kaolin) that absorbs sebum. "Oil-control" foundations simply contain more of these substances to absorb higher concentrations of oil. That does not necessarily mean they are also oil-free—although they may be. You have to check the label.

Oil-free foundations usually come in a liquid form that is easy to apply and lasts well on the skin. They may also be formulated as simple shake lotions—with pigmented talc suspended in water and solvents. These evaporate quickly once the makeup is applied, leaving a thin layer of powder on the face. These somewhat old-fashioned foundations do not provide a lot of coverage, but they do reduce shine, and their simple formulations and minimal ingredients can make them a good choice for women with sensitive skin.

COLOR AND CAMOUFLAGE

According to makeup artist Bobbi Brown, creator of Bobbi Brown Cosmetics, women with acne make several characteristic errors when it comes to foundation. "The biggest mistake they make is that they buy the thickest, most cakey makeup they can find to cover their acne. And then they apply it so heavily that it draws attention to the blemishes, instead of taking attention away. Also, they usually pick a pinky or beigey tone that has no relationship to the skin on their body, so the whole thing just looks like a thick mask. Foundation should look like skin. If you put it on and it doesn't look like skin, it's the wrong foundation."

Color is crucial, says Brown, who advises a neutral color, without orange, red, pink, or blue undertones. "You need a foundation that matches your skin exactly. And it should be yellow-toned—whether you have light skin or dark." With very rare exceptions (for example, some Native Americans or Pacific Islanders, who have reddish undertones in their skin), most people, whatever their skin color or racial background, have skin with yellow undertones because the skin pigment melanin is yellow.

"Also, all makeup turns a little more orange on oily skin, so you don't want to start out with anything reddish or orangey," says Brown. "Yellow is the key. For foundation, concealer, and powder."

Brown recommends trying out colors at a department store. "Because color is the hardest thing to get right. So even if you don't have a lot of money, I suggest going to a department store where you can allow yourself time and actually test the colors. The way to do that is to try it on the side of your cheek, then turn your head from side to side and see if it blends in. In most stores, you'll have to step outside to get the right light. If the foundation matches your skin exactly, you've got the right color. If you look at it and say, 'Oh my God, this makes me look too yellow,' that doesn't mean it's really too yellow, it just means it's too dark. So go back and get a lighter shade."

Concealers to mask blemishes should match your foundation. Never use your undereye concealer on a blemish. It is usually a shade lighter than your foundation, and if you put a light color on a blemish, it's going to make it stand out more. The whole idea is to match your skin and your foundation.

If you are using a medicated spot treatment on a blemish, it should go under the foundation. But concealers used for camouflage do a better job if they're on top. "I do the foundation first," says Brown. "That provides a lot of coverage itself, sometimes all you need. If not, then I go back with a little brush, and I kind of paint on the concealer with little dots. Just wherever the red is."

MAKEUP "MIGRATION"

In a small study published in 2001 in the *Journal of the American Academy of Dermatology*, Wake Forest University's Draelos set out to discover what happens to makeup when it gets on the skin, and solve the mystery of where it goes as it disappears. She examined twelve women—four with dry skin, four with normal skin, and four with oily skin—every hour over an eight-hour period, under a high-powered video microscope.

She learned that within two hours of application, makeup pigment particles began to migrate, heading into the follicles (as well as into facial folds and wrinkles). Makeup on the women with oily skin migrated the fastest, "floating" pigment particles into the pores. Draelos speculated that this may explain why foundations that are labeled "non-comedogenic" and "non-acnegenic" may cause acneiform eruptions in some women. (Most people who experience adverse reactions to foundations experience follicular papules and pustules within forty-eight hours.)

Interestingly, the calamine lotion–like "shake makeups" stayed put the longest. Liquid foundations migrated less rapidly than thick cream/powder ones. But whatever the formulation, after four hours of wear, all of the foundations had degraded to a point where they no longer provided an even film over the face—which goes a long way toward explaining why by lunchtime your face may look like it just rolled out of bed.

You can retard foundation creep a little by preparing your skin before you apply makeup, with one of the oil-absorbing agents, and by setting it with face powder. Powder helps makeup stay in place both by preventing movement and by absorbing the perspiration and sebum that act to float the pigments away. Face powder also helps keep sunscreen, which is also lifted off the skin by perspiration and sebum, on the face and working longer.

"Make sure you put powder on with a puff," advises Brown. "Not a brush, but a velour puff. Like those old-fashioned ones you've seen in the movies. Cotton balls get stuff all over the place. Sponges are porous. And a brush just kind of dusts it on. You need a puff with a velvety surface because that will put the powder where it's needed, and then it will really grip the face. You want to really press it around the nose, and around the chin—the areas where you need it. And use tinted powder; translucent just makes your skin look ashy and white. There needs to be a just a little tint to it so it looks natural."

Be judicious about repowdering during the day; the powder can absorb so much sebum that it turns into a sludgy-looking mess. Blot up oil instead with one of the oil-blotting papers that many cosmetic companies make for that very purpose. If you do want to dab a little powder on your nose, blot your skin first with the paper. And I know this sounds a little odd (even off-putting), but one of the best ways to arrest shine, if you don't have any of the special tissues, is to use a piece of one of those paper toilet seat covers found in ladies' rest rooms. Unlike a Kleenex or a paper towel, it's got just the right texture to sop up oil without depositing little bits of paper or tissue fuzz on your face.

Once you've got the foundation, the concealer, and the powder all down, you can pretty much do whatever you like with the rest of your makeup. But bear in mind that blushers and other colored makeup with built-in shimmer or sparkle tend to catch the light and draw attention to any skin imperfections. Brown suggests using makeup to focus attention on your eyes or lips—whichever you regard as the best of those two features—as a means of drawing attention away from any flaws in your complexion.

"My advice always is to get your attention away from whatever bugs you," she says. "If you have acne, cover up your skin as well as you can, then do your eyes or use a pretty lipstick, and don't worry about it. I've had women come up to me and say, 'Look at this horrible scar' or 'this awful blemish,' and you know what? I never noticed it, because I was looking at their beautiful eyes or their wonderful hair. Women all tend to look at the worst thing on themselves and think it's all everybody else sees. The truth is, that's not what other people see. The only person who sees your worst thing first is yourself. I really believe that other people see a person's best things first."

Chapter Twelve

◄◇►

Acne and Your Children

BACK WHEN HE WAS ELEVEN YEARS OLD and in the sixth grade, my oldest son came to me one day and surprised me by asking how he could keep from getting acne. At the time he had what appeared to be totally unblemished skin. But on close inspection, he could detect a few pinpoint-sized pimples on his nose. Even more significantly (in his mind), he had already begun to see some of his classmates break out with obvious red bumps.

"I don't *ever* want that to happen to me," he said, shuddering. "It's so . . . *ugly*."

Well. As wounded as I was by the latter sentiment, I could certainly relate to the former. After years of battling breakouts myself, I didn't want my child to suffer anywhere near the same fate. Certainly any mother—any parent—who has ever had serious acne must feel a similar desire to spare her offspring the myriad consequences of acne.

It is a legitimate concern. Although doctors have not definitively pinned down the precise genetic links, acne does run in families. If you have ever had significant acne, your children have at least a 50-50 chance of suffering from it as well. Moreover, if it shows up, chances are it will probably occur in about the same manner in your child as it did in you. Dermatologists seeing young acne patients for the first time often eye the parents' skin for clues about the potential course of the disease in their children. What they see in terms of scarring on the parent can serve as a remarkably accurate predictor of how serious the acne is likely to be in the child.

But it doesn't have to be. An assertive, proactive approach can help to ensure that even a child earmarked by genetic fate for terrible acne need not suffer the worst manifestations of the disease itself, or the disfiguring scars it is destined to leave behind.

"We have a much more aggressive attitude today," emphasizes Munich's Professor Gerd Plewig. "We treat acne much earlier than we did before, and of course we have much better drugs than we did in the past. So the very severe cases? The very bad scars? We don't have to see them anymore. They don't have to happen."

ACNE IN INFANCY

Acne can occur at any age. In fact, facial breakouts are almost as common in the first year of life as they are in puberty. They appear in two forms. Newborn (or "neonatal") acne crops up at birth or within a couple of weeks afterward. What is known as "infantile" acne shows up later, after three months or more.

Neonatal acne is by far the more common of the two. "If you go into the nursery of any hospital and take a good look at every newborn there, you'll probably see something that looks like acne on at least half of them," says pediatric dermatologist Howard Pride, assistant professor of pediatrics and dermatology at Pennsylvania State University.

Seeing a face full of red bumps on your cherished infant can, of course, completely freak you out if you have ever had troublesome acne yourself. ("Is that *acne*? On my *baby*!?)

Happily, in most cases, there's nothing to worry about. Pediatricians rarely give neonatal acne a second thought, and they reassure parents that the breakouts will vanish within a few months. In fact, as many as half of newborns with what appears to be acne are afflicted instead with minor skin eruptions that merely look like acne.

Little white bumps—milia—are very common on infants, and typically disappear within a couple of weeks. Sometimes acne-like pimples on a baby are the result of skin-irritating agents, such as an ingredient in an oil or lotion. And about 3 percent of all newborns develop a form of folliculitis known as neonatal cephalic pustulosis, caused by a yeast-like organism called *Malassezia sympodialis*. *Malassezia* is one of the many organisms that live unseen and unheeded on everyone's skin. But some babies have a reaction to it and develop small acne-like bumps, which doctors treat with a topical anti-yeast medication, such as ketoconazole. As the babies mature, their skin becomes less sensitive to the yeast, and the breakouts clear up.

Some 15 to 20 percent of babies do break out in a form of true acne: red bumps and pustules—sometimes mixed with tiny whiteheads and blackheads—over the cheeks, and sometimes on the chin and forehead. They are apparently caused by androgens acting on the sebaceous follicles in much the same way that they do in acne-prone adolescents and adults. Doctors used to assume (and many still tell parents) that the offending hormones were acquired from the mother, either in the womb or through breast-feeding. Now they recognize that the acne-stimulating androgens are in large part the baby's own, pumped out by the oversized adrenal glands that all infants have at birth. In baby boys, the testes produce additional androgens.

The result is that newborns briefly experience what is known as a "hormonal milieu" similar to that of adolescents. Oily skin and acne can be a result.

Neonatal acne is rarely cause for concern. It seldom lasts long. It does not leave scars, and, thus far, researchers have not found any evidence that newborns with acne are any more likely than their clear-skinned peers to suffer serious breakouts in adolescence or beyond. Most doctors simply recommend waiting it out. By about three months, an infant's adrenal glands shrink to the size they will remain until puberty. Sebum production plummets, and the skin takes on the magically silken quality we think of when we picture a baby's skin.

However, if a baby has obvious comedones or severe inflammation, dermatologists may apply topical kerolytic ointments (such as salicylic acid), mild benzoyl peroxide preparations, or even a retinoid. Surprisingly, babies treated with Retin-A or other topical retinoids rarely experience the irritation that older children, teenagers, and adults frequently do, possibly because infant skin is better hydrated and less sun-damaged than that of teens or adults.

CHILDHOOD ACNE

What doctors call infantile (or "early-childhood") acne is far less common than neonatal acne, and it is usually much more serious. Unlike newborn acne, it is often linked to family history, and it may herald an increased risk of developing severe acne as a teen. Infantile acne can appear at any age from three months to three years or older; six to twelve months is common. Characterized by blackheads, whiteheads, and inflamed papules and pustules, especially on the cheeks, it can last anywhere from six months to three years or more, and it may leave obvious scars.

"It is very aggressive, and scarring is a real worry," says Pride, who stresses that acne in a child between the age of six months and eight or nine years may indicate another, underlying medical condition. "Acne in children this age is not normal and ought to raise a red flag."

Early-childhood acne tends to appear somewhat more frequently in boys than in girls; doctors believe that it may be related to premature secretion of androgens from the testes. Particularly severe cases call for medical testing in order to determine if there is an underlying endocrine disorder, such as congenital adrenal hyperplasia, a condition in which the adrenal glands are abnormally enlarged.

"However, if there is a true hormonal abnormality—if very high levels of androgens are present—it would be very unusual if acne were the only sign," says Pride. "For instance, you would likely also see out-of-the-ordinary growth, or, in males, larger than normal testicles."

Whatever the root cause (and however another medical specialist, such as a pediatrician or endocrinologist, may treat it), dermatologists address the breakouts of childhood acne much as they do those of adolescents, commonly with topical retinoids and antibacterial agents, such as benzoyl peroxide. Severe or persistent inflammation may call for an oral antibiotic, typically erythromycin. (Tetracycline should not be given to children this young because it causes discoloration of developing teeth.)

If there are nodules and cysts that do not respond to treatment, particularly if the child is developing scars, doctors may turn to Accutane—an admittedly disquieting prospect for parents who may be anxious about the drug's potential side effects.

"Accutane for a child this young makes us all a little nervous," says Pride. "You do worry about side effects, and there is a concern about whether it will cause skeletal changes. But Accutane is a very reasonable thing to prescribe if the acne is severe and scarring, and if you can't get it under control any other way." He adds that young patients who receive Accutane therapy for severe forms of a congenital skin condition called ichthyosis do not suffer serious side effects from long-term use of the drug—evidence that it also should not harm young acne patients.

ADOLESCENCE

Adolescence is, of course, the time when you expect your child to get acne. But it may appear at a much younger age than you anticipated—as early as eight in some girls; at nine or ten in some boys.

Acne in the preteen years is typically one of the signs of what is known as adrenarche, which means the maturation of the adrenal glands. Adrenarche is the first of two stages of puberty; it is sometimes referred to as "prepuberty," and it has noticeable effects on the skin: underarm odor (a result of maturing sweat glands), perhaps the first wisps of genital and underarm hair, and increased levels of sebum. In acne-prone kids, there may also be whiteheads, blackheads, and even small pimples.

The second stage of puberty, sometimes called true puberty, involves maturation of the ovaries in girls and of the testes in boys. This brings on new waves of hormones that can stimulate new acne breakouts, or aggravate an existing case.

At whatever age it appears, it is prudent to take acne seriously and to try to keep on top of it with appropriate treatment for whatever stage it's in. "We can't prevent acne, but we can keep it at a very low flame," says Plewig. "Especially if we start topical treatment in very young children—at eleven or twelve, a very early age. Topical retinoids if the child is at risk.

Sometimes we even start systemic treatment with Accutane at this stage—especially if both parents have had serious acne."

Typically, however, early treatment is much less aggressive. "When a mother comes in with a teen who's got active acne, and asks, 'By the way, what do I do for the ten-year-old at home who's starting to get a few blackheads?' I tell her to get salicylic acid," says acne expert Alan Shalita. "Salicylic acid, of course, is not tremendously effective, but it will help with the very mild cases in young kids—if they'll use it."

If they'll use it. Which is far from certain, especially if their acne is mild, says Fairfax, Virginia, pediatric dermatologist Robert Silverman, clinical associate professor of pediatrics and dermatology at Georgetown University, who explains that it is not always easy to get a child or teen to comply with any acne treatment regimen. "If they don't think they've got much of a problem to begin with, then they're probably not going to stick with it," he warns.

It can be especially difficult to get a youngster to appreciate that all acne treatment is essentially preventive. "I try to get the concept across by telling them it's like brushing your teeth. You brush your teeth to prevent cavities; you use acne medicine to keep from getting big pustules. But, you know, a lot of these kids don't brush their teeth every night, either. Parents can beat their heads against the wall, but if the child doesn't see the acne as a problem, it's not going to get done. They'll only do it when they're ready. Of course, if a child has severe, scarring inflammatory acne, you hope they'll be ready."

Silverman advises keeping children's and teens' regimens as simple as possible. "The more things you add, the less compliance you get," he notes. "What I tell them to do for mild acne is wash their faces two times a day with a salicylic acid soap, using just their hands. You don't want them to use something rough, like a washcloth, because the more they rub and scrub, the more damage they'll do. The soaps are only mildly effective—at best—but regular cleansing, I think, gets kids in the mood to go to the other treatment they need, whether it's a topical retinoid or something else. If they have any inflammation, any papules or pustules, I'll have them use benzoyl peroxide—just 2.5 percent, which is as useful as 5 or 10 percent, but not as irritating."

That, in fact, is almost precisely the acne-fighting regimen my own son started following at eleven, after we rummaged through my stockpile of over-the-counter acne medicines to find a few he could live with. By process of elimination (that is to say, he eliminated any product contained in what he judged to be "feminine" packaging) and a little trial and error, we unearthed a few acne fighters he liked. One was Oxy Balance Facial Cleansing Wash, a 2 percent salicylic acid cleanser in a gender-neutral red, white, and blue bottle. Another was Proactiv Repairing Lotion—a mild 2.5 percent benzoyl peroxide lotion. He added a sulfur-based spot treatment called Acnomel, for the few occasional blemishes that did break through.

And . . . it worked! Three years later, at fourteen—the age I had been when my acne exploded—he was still following the same basic regime, and was still virtually blemish-free. I was jubilant, figuring I had saved my child from my own awful adolescent fate. Unfortunately, it's not that simple—as I learned when I crowed about my success to Dr. Pride of Penn State.

"If a kid is fated to get bad acne, early treatment is not going to totally head it off at the pass," he informed me. The most likely explanation for my son's acne-free early teenage complexion, he explained, was that he simply lucked out and did not inherit my much more severely acne-prone skin. Or maybe it wasn't going to appear until he was older.

Which is not to say that the Oxy Balance Wash and the Proactiv Lotion had no effect at all. They probably did a fine job of keeping mild breakouts at bay. But my son would have needed (and may still need as he gets older) stronger medicine, such as topical retinoids along with a benzoyl peroxide preparation or antibiotics, for a more severe problem.

The important thing is to keep on top of acne—at whatever stage it is in—and never adopt a wait-and-see attitude, which can allow things to get out of hand. "Many, many parents still tell their children, 'Just wait until it goes away,' " says Plewig. "You must never do that."

Then again, notes Silverman, you also have to be realistic.

"Parents who have had bad acne themselves are generally quite concerned, and they will bring in their kids very early— even when the kids don't have much showing on their faces and maybe haven't even noticed anything themselves. But you really can't keep teens completely clear and have their skin looking like they're seven years old. Acne can be managed. It can be treated so that you don't have the severe inflammation and the bad scarring. But you're not going to totally stop the process."

"There is only one thing that can really alter the natural course of acne," adds Pride. "And that's Accutane."

ACCUTANE AND YOUR CHILD

There may be no more difficult moment for parents of a child with serious acne than when it looks as if Accutane (isotretinoin) is the next logical step. Even if you know you would feel confident using it yourself, should you need it, you may find yourself apprehensive about the prospect of allowing your child to take it. Indeed, a quick review of Accutane's possible side effects (pages 93-99) would give any parent pause.

A simple Internet search can terrify you. Type "Accutane"

into any online search engine, and in five minutes you can find enough frightening anecdotal information about the drug's alleged links to suicide in young people to convince you that allowing your child to take it is tantamount to letting him play Russian roulette.

But statistically speaking, the risk appears to be infinitesimal. Papers presented at the American Academy of Dermatology's annual meetings in 2001 and 2002 compared the numbers of reported suicides of patients taking Accutane with the general suicide statistics in the United States, and found that the rate of suicide in Accutane patients is far less than that among the total population.

According to the available figures, there are, in total, some 30,000 suicides per year in the United States, a rate of 11.4 per 100,000. Compared to that, the reported rate of suicides among isotretinoin users is 1.8 in 100,000 users. Dermatologists also take note of the fact that the rate of suicide among young people in general is high. (In the United States, there are some 6,000 suicides per year in the fifteen- to twenty-four-year-old age group, making suicide the third leading cause of death among young adults in America.)

The median age of the thirty-seven Accutane users reported to have killed themselves between the years 1982 and 2000 was seventeen years old. Extrapolating from the number of suicides of fifteen- to nineteen-year-olds in the general population and the number in that age range who were using Accutane, the number of Accutane users who might have been expected to commit suicide would have been nine times as high as it was.

Opponents of the acne drug dispute these figures, saying the number of suicide deaths among Accutane users reported to the Food and Drug Administration—keepers of the statistics in cases like this—are lower than the actual numbers who have died. They further charge that drug makers, and perhaps some dermatologists, have failed to report some of the cases they should have. The dispute has most recently come to national attention because of some high-profile cases.

The most notable of these was the suicide death of Michigan congressman Bart Stupak's seventeen-year-old-son, B.J., an acne sufferer, in the spring of 2000. At the time, the youth had been taking Accutane for several months, and his father came to believe that his death was linked to the drug's reported psychiatric side effects. Congressman Stupak has since campaigned vigorously for renewed FDA scrutiny of isotretinoin's psychological side effects, and his is the most prominent voice calling for tighter restrictions on the drug.

Dermatologists reply that Accutane is invaluable because it controls severe acne in adolescents as no other treatment can. They point out that many young people with disfiguring acne who do *not* take Accutane often suffer from severe depression, which itself can lead to suicide. For these deeply unhappy young people, Accutane can have life-transforming effects. "Accutane is a fantastic, wonderful medicine that *saves* children's lives, because it saves their psyches," exclaims dermatologist Laurie Polis, who once suffered from terrible acne herself and says she wouldn't hesitate to prescribe it for her own children if they needed it. "It is the greatest innovation ever in dermatology. Thank *God* for Accutane!"

Every dermatologist I've ever asked about the subject expresses similar feelings. (That's not to say there *aren't* any dermatologists who would not give it to their own children. It's just that I haven't met any.) But grieving parents of Accutane users who have taken their own lives or who have experienced profound emotional changes while on the drug are just as heartfelt in their conviction that it represents a genuine danger to young people.

There is no easy answer for parents who are apprehensive about Accutane, concedes dermatologist and psychologist Richard Fried, who has examined the available medical histories of known suicide victims whose deaths were linked to the drug. Along with other experts who have similarly investigated these case histories over the years, he has concluded that most of the victims had psychiatric symptoms indicating they were at risk for suicide prior to taking the medicine, and the fact that they were on Accutane at the time of their deaths was coincidental.

"That's not to say that any one person won't experience an idiosyncratic harmful reaction from any drug. But we have now had two generations of experience with Accutane, and while it may well have produced some psychiatric side effects in some small number of patients, there has never been any convincing medical or scientific evidence that it has caused a suicide."

Fried, Pride, Silverman, and other pediatric experts all emphasize that it is vital for parents contemplating Accutane therapy for a child to seek out a dermatologist who is experienced both in prescribing the drug and in monitoring patients who are on it, and to insist on a detailed and thorough discussion of all the potential risks and benefits.

"I tell parents it's like the scales of justice," says Fried. "On the one hand, you have a infinitesimal, unproven risk. On the other, you have a disfiguring disease that is affecting your child now and will leave scars that will last the rest of his life. I know that making decisions on behalf of your children is one of the hardest things you will ever have to do as a parent. But I have to say that for a kid not to have to walk into a classroom, or a social event, and be covered with these terrible skin lesions, to have him grow up not experiencing all of the pain that serious acne can inflict, that is a very fair thing to owe your child."

Chapter Thirteen

———◇———

Scars and Scar Revision

IN ONE OF MY MOST VIVID MEMORIES of talking to another woman with acne, I am sitting in the Washington, D.C., office of laser surgeon Tina Alster with one of her patients. She is a beautiful woman in her early thirties, but her cheeks and chin are densely covered with small shallow scars. Their edges catch the light and cast tiny shadows, creating a harsh little moonscape of tiny craters and chasms. There doesn't seem to be a square quarter-inch of normal-looking skin on her face from below her eyes to above her jawline. I lean in for a closer look, and she peers back at me.

We're comparing notes. I have fewer scars, but they're much deeper. She has many, many more, but they are extremely shallow. Secretly, I'm thanking my lucky stars. I have despaired for years over my own acne scars, but I am suddenly filled with gratitude that there aren't more of them and that I at least have large areas of normal-looking skin. For perhaps the first time ever, I'm gaining a little honest perspective. Things could definitely be worse.

Then again, very shallow scarring such as hers seems a much better prospect for skin resurfacing—much more likely to smooth out and fade into insignificance under the laser's beam. I tell her that, and she starts to cry.

"Oh, God, I hope that's right," she says, weeping. "I used to think that having acne was the worst thing that ever happened to me. But no matter how bad it gets, you always have hope. You know that *someday* it's going to go away. And you think it will be over then. But *this*? There's just no hope."

ABOUT ACNE SCARS

Happily, acne scars are not truly hopeless. But they do present a difficult challenge to the surgeon's skills because they are as destructive to the physical structure of the skin as their appearance is to the psyche.

Human skin is composed of three layers. At the surface is the epidermis. The dermis, which lies just below, consists of a meshwork of protein strands (collagen and elastin) that look very much like the threads that make up woven cloth. The bottom layer is the subcutis, or fatty layer.

Acne scars are caused by inflamed lesions that destroy a portion of the dermis and its collagen network. Occasionally, the skin responds by overproducing new collagen, creating a raised, or "hypertrophic," scar. More commonly, the collagen grows back only partially or not at all, leaving a depressed, or "atrophic," scar.

Depending on the severity and extent of the inflammatory destruction, atrophic acne scars range in contour from shallow undulating depressions and saucer-like indentations, to deep pits and jagged-edged craters that make the skin look as if it has been jabbed with an ice pick or other sharp instrument. Some, called "full-thickness" scars, extend all the way through the dermis into the fatty subcutis.

Frequently, atrophic scars are bound down—tethered like a balloon held to earth by ropes—to the tissues below them with bands of collagen that run straight into the subcutaneous tissue. These scars tend to become increasingly evident as a person ages and gradually loses subcutaneous fat. The skin sags, but parts of it remain hitched to the underlying tissues by the fibrous bands.

Few acne scars can be completely eliminated by any means, which is why experienced doctors typically speak in terms of "revising" them or "reducing" their appearance, rather than "erasing" or "eradicating" them. The most common approach is to resurface the skin—by such techniques as laser ablation, chemical peels, or dermabrasion. But most acne scars penetrate far below the level where skin can safely be removed. Only the most minor, superficial scars can actually be expunged. Most can only be reduced in size and depth.

"Some doctors say you can expect to get up to 80 percent improvement in acne scars with resurfacing, but I always say it's just in the 50 percent range or less," comments dermatologic surgeon Harold Brody, clinical professor of dermatology at Atlanta's Emory University, and author of two highly regarded textbooks on skin resurfacing and chemical peels. "You just can't get 80 percent improvement with resurfacing alone. Especially if the scars are big or if they're full thickness, 50 percent is about the best you can hope for."

For optimum results, says Brody, depressed acne scars generally require both resurfacing and additional treatment, often by injecting or implanting cosmetic filler material such as collagen beneath the depression to raise it up. "That's when you can get 80 percent improvement. When you both resurface and use some sort of filler."

Resurfacing and filling, however, are appropriate only for shallow, undulating, or soft-sided scars. Neither method works well to reduce ice-pick scars, or other sharp-sided, punched-out-looking pits. These are too deep to be more than marginally affected by resurfacing. And they are lined with tough, fibrous scar tissue that cannot be displaced by either injected or implanted fillers. "The only thing that works for them is surgical excision," says Brody. "You have to take them out first, then resurface the skin."

You can get a rough idea of what type of treatment your own scars may need in any given location by using your fingers to stretch the skin there and see how the scars react. Pulling the skin taut will make shallow or soft-sided scars almost or totally disappear; those scars generally can be corrected with resurfacing and fillers. Scars that you can't stretch out by pulling on the skin (called nondistensible scars) generally require surgical excision.

SURGICAL EXCISION

For large, nondistensible scars, some doctors use a method called subcision, inserting a beveled needle under the scar and moving it back and forth to cut the fibrous strands of collagen that are holding it down. "This can be useful for some scars, but there are trade-offs," says dermatologic surgeon Richard Glogau, clinical professor of dermatology at the University of California in San Francisco. "You get a fair amount of bruising and discoloration with subcision, which can take a long time to heal. Also, it's unpredictable. You can bust up that fibrotic tissue, but the fibrosis reestablishes itself fairly readily and it can wind up looking just like it did before."

Another common means of removal is called punch excision, typically used for ice-pick scars. The scar is punched out of the skin with a biopsy punch instrument that looks a little like an apple corer. This leaves a tiny cylindrical hole. Depending on its size and location, the cavity is then either closed with a small suture, or filled in with what is known as a punch graft—a plug of skin taken from behind the patient's ear.

In a related technique, called punch elevation, a punch is used to cut the scar loose from its surroundings. Then it is lifted up flush with the skin surface and left in place to heal. In some cases, if the scars are large, or if there are several in a row, an entire section of skin may be punched out or excised. For badly scarred skin, a doctor may have to punch out hundreds of little scars—a time-consuming and labor-intensive effort. "But nothing else is going to help those scars," says Brody.

Punch grafts, excisions, and elevations often leave new scars—small circular or linear lines—that may be resurfaced six to eight weeks later. A newer approach, particularly if there is extensive scarring, is to punch out or excise scars at the same time as laser resurfacing or dermabrasion, so that the skin surface and the small incisions will all heal together, leaving much less conspicuous lines of demarcation between excision areas and the surrounding skin.

RESURFACING AND COLLAGEN REMODELING

Skin resurfacing works by removing layers of skin to create a wound. The wound heals by generating new cells that create a smoother, less-flawed surface. Two healing mechanisms come into play. One, reepithelializing, is the replacement of the skin's upper surface, the epidermis. The other, collagen remodeling, is a change in the collagen network of the middle layer, the dermis.

The dermis consists of a thin upper ("papillary") portion composed of loosely woven collagen strands, and a lower ("reticular") portion made up of dense, thick bundles of collagen. Collagen remodeling occurs as a result of resurfacing techniques that remove or damage the papillary dermis, and at least some portion of the reticular dermis. Collagen-producing cells (called fibroblasts) repair the damage by creating new collagen strands that are more abundant and regular in shape than before. This provides a new support structure that stretches and "plumps up" the epidermis, much in the way a wrinkled bedsheet is stretched smooth by a firm new mattress.

Acne scars can be substantially improved only by resurfacing methods that injure the dermis sufficiently to promote collagen remodeling. Although sometimes touted as a means of treating acne scars, the exfoliating glycolic acid peels or microdermabrasion treatments performed in salons or spas do not do this. Neither do what are known as "superficial epidermal peels," medical procedures that employ chemicals or abrasives to remove the epidermis along with any superficial flaws (moderate sun damage, irregular pigmentation) it might contain.

Superficial peels are also sometimes promoted as scar treatments, particularly when performed in a series of four, six, eight, or more sessions. But while they may well initially make acne-scarred skin look better, the effects are typically due to temporary skin swelling. Repeated superficial peels may also stimulate the growth of some new collagen in the dermis, theoretically plumping up overlying scars. But according to Brody, "Even if they do cause a little bit of collagen to build up beneath the epidermis, there is no way it translates to a clinical result [i.e., a result you can see] for acne scars. It just doesn't. To affect acne scars, you have to have deep, dermal collagen remodeling."

This occurs, to a modest extent, with what are categorized as medium-depth peels, which remove the entire papillary dermis and a thin, upper portion of the reticular dermis. Medium-depth peels are among the most popular of all cosmetic procedures, widely used to improve the appearance of wrinkles, pigmentation irregularities, and other signs of aging or sun damage.

The most common medium-depth procedures are chemical peels, in which a chemical agent is applied directly to the skin to destroy one or more of its layers at a time. Doctors typically employ a chemical called trichloroacetic acid (TCA), often in combination with other materials that enhance penetration or depth control. (Proprietary name-brand peels such as the Accupeel or the Obagi Blue Peel are medium-depth TCA peels with added bells and whistles.)

Medium-depth peels have only a moderate effect on acne scars, and only under optimal circumstances, according to Brody. "A medium-depth peel, when properly done by a physician who's trained in it, can remodel acne scarring and achieve about a 20 percent improvement." But many medium peels, he warns, produce virtually no visible results at all. "This is the least effective of the resurfacing procedures for acne scarring."

DEEP PEELS FOR VISIBLE RESULTS

Resurfacing for acne scars is really the province of deep laser resurfacing and dermabrasion, which remove skin tissue all the way down into the midreticular dermis to promote extensive collagen remodeling. (The deep chemical peels sometimes used on fair-skinned people to treat wrinkles or sun damage tend to cause complete or near-complete loss of skin pigment, and are not appropriate for acne scarring, says Brody.)

Both laser resurfacing and dermabrasion are serious surgical procedures that involve long healing periods and a certain amount of risk. They are highly technique-dependent, meaning that the results are directly proportionate to the skill and experience of the surgeon who performs the delicate balancing act of going deeply enough into the skin to remove as much of the scar as possible and stimulate as much collagen remodeling as feasible, while stopping just short of compromising the skin's ability to heal properly.

Penetrating below the midreticular dermis imperils the skin's ability to generate a normal new surface, and may damage or destroy pigment-producing melanocytes, causing permanent changes in skin color. Aggressive resurfacing also can so ravage the collagen-producing fibroblasts that they can no longer produce normal collagen.

Deep peels can be safely performed only on the face because facial skin is relatively thick and contains the body's most abundant collection of pilosebaceous units—the structures that are critical for regenerating a new epidermis. (Intact epidermal cells inside the follicle generate new cells that travel up and migrate over the skin to create a new surface.)

Other parts of the body heal more slowly than the face and are at much greater risk of scarring or other complications from resurfacing. In general, this means that neither resurfacing lasers nor dermabrasion can be safely used on the neck or on the back, where many people have acne scars. Doctors usually treat those areas with milder chemical peels that improve the texture of the skin and make it more similar in color to the more aggressively treated areas on the face. Scars on the neck or back may also be improved by treatment with nonablative lasers (discussed below), which help to restore underlying collagen.

Both laser resurfacing and dermabrasion have an impact on the skin's pigment-producing melanocytes, and both can produce changes in skin color—either browning (hyperpigmentation) from melanocytes reacting to the injury, or skin lightening (hypopigmentation) if the melanocytes have been damaged in such a way that they produce less pigment.

Dark-skinned patients are most likely to experience pigmentation difficulties, but anyone's skin color may be affected by resurfacing. It is very common for laser-treated skin of any color to darken and turn brown, starting two to four weeks after the surgery. Caught early, postsurgical hyperpigmentation can be arrested with topical creams containing skin-lightening chemicals such as hydroquinone. A doctor may also prescribe light chemical peels or exfoliating treatments with glycolic or azelaic acid. Without such treatment, it can take up to a year for the skin gradually to return to its original hue. (That, by the way, presumes you've strictly avoided the sun; healing skin exposed to damaging ultraviolet light may never return to its original color.)

Laser Resurfacing

Laser resurfacing is today's most common resurfacing procedure for acne scarring. It is typically performed with either a carbon dioxide (CO_2) laser, so called because the laser beam passes through a chamber filled with carbon dioxide gas, or with an Erbium:YAG laser (named for the crystal through which the beam passes).

The CO_2 laser's precision, ease of use, and collagen-remodeling prowess revolutionized skin resurfacing in the 1990s. And expert laser surgeons still regard treatment with the pulsed or scanned carbon dioxide laser as the gold standard of skin resurfacing. "There still isn't anything else that can really match it," says leading laser specialist Tina Alster, of Georgetown University, who has written several textbooks on laser surgery and has worked with many different dermatologic lasers.

She cautions that the CO_2 laser's impressive attributes come at a steep price for patients: a painful and lengthy healing period, prolonged redness (most patients look as if they have a bad sunburn for months), and lingering changes in skin color. The CO_2 laser is particularly hard on dark skin, inevitably causing hyperpigmentation in Asian, African American, and Hispanic patients. "You can counteract these pigment changes," says Alster. "But you have to know how, and I strongly advise dark-skinned patients to be particularly careful in seeking out a laser surgeon who is experienced in treating dark skin and managing its side effects."

The Erbium laser is regarded as a kinder, gentler alternative to the CO_2 laser. Due to the different characteristics of its beam, it produces less heating in the dermis, so treated skin heals more rapidly, and with less redness. The Erbium laser also has a less traumatic effect on melanocytes.

The trade-off is less collagen remodeling. So any improvement in acne scars treated with the Erbium laser will likely be less pronounced than that from CO_2 resurfacing. Laser specialists sometimes use both on the same patient, making a single pass over the face with the CO_2 laser, then completing the procedure with the Erbium laser. This minimizes the potential side effects of CO_2 resurfacing, while still taking advantage of some of its superior collagen remodeling capacity.

DERMABRASION

The oldest of all resurfacing methods, dermabrasion was largely eclipsed by the laser craze of the mid-1990s, as dermatologists by the droves mothballed their old dermabrasion equipment to embrace the new technology. Many dermatologists frankly hated dermabrasion, a horrifically bloody procedure in which a rapidly rotating, abrasive metal wheel is used like a carpenter's sander to mechanically remove layers of skin. Because of the blood, it is very difficult for a surgeon to determine how the treatment is progressing and how deeply the skin has been abraded. It takes an artist's touch to get the best results; ham-handed technique can produce an unnaturally contoured skin surface as wavy as unevenly sanded wood.

Louisiana's Dr. John Yarborough, of Tulane University, regarded by other dermatologists as one of the modern masters of dermabrasion, trained as a concert pianist before turning to medicine, and says that people have often speculated that he owes his exceptional dexterity with dermabrasion to his many years of practice at the keyboard.

According to Yarborough, dermabrasion's mechanical action is intrinsically more suitable for resurfacing acne scars than the light from a laser. "You can really break up the base of those fibrous scars with dermabrasion." Moreover, although the procedure is appallingly gory, he maintains that it is actually less painful in the long run than laser resurfacing, and that the skin heals much faster and with less impact on its natural color. "I believe that's because dermabrasion is primarily a mechanical injury and laser is a thermal injury. Every one of us has skinned our knees, and we don't have any marks; but if you are standing in front of a stove and it splatters grease on your hands, it takes the pigment right out. And it takes forever to heal."

Brody also gives the edge to dermabrasion for acne scars, and notes that the technique has experienced something of a renaissance. "I increasingly now choose dermabrasion over the laser for acne scars. In fact, I'll bet that today there are 65 to 75 percent fewer laser procedures for acne scars than there were in 1995," he says. "Dermabrasion is more economical, the healing time is shorter, and it's not as fraught with so much loss of pigment."

Dermabrasion's chief drawback is the fact that it has become increasingly difficult to find an experienced, proficient practitioner to do it. "I think it may be something of a dying art," says Yarborough ruefully. "We used to have scads of people coming down here to learn how to do it. But we don't anymore."

NONABLATIVE LASER "RESURFACING"

So-called "nonablative" lasers—commercially known by such evocative names as "CoolTouch" and "Smoothbeam"—send their light through the epidermis to plump up the skin from the inside. The laser beam passes harmlessly though the skin surface and is absorbed by the tissues in the dermis, creating heat that stimulates collagen remodeling. A device built into the hand piece simultaneously sprays the skin surface with a cooling liquid to lessen the patient's discomfort and to prevent heat from injuring the underside of the epidermis. As the dermal tissue recovers from the heat damage, the collagen contracts and tightens, smoothing defects in the skin above.

Nonablative laser surgery, and a similar technique called photo-rejuvenation, have become increasingly popular as bloodless "face-lifting" treatments for fine or moderate wrinkling. And because they have little effect on the pigment-producing cells of the epidermis, they present an attractive option for patients with dark skin. But the results are far more subtle than those produced by either the CO_2 or the Erbium laser. Multiple treatments (typically three to five sessions, spaced four to six weeks apart) are required to achieve noticeable effects. Some surgeons also use nonablative lasers six to eighteen months following conventional laser resurfacing to enhance or help maintain the collagen remodeling effects of the ablative lasers.

This is very much an evolving technology, and its effects on acne scarring remain problematic, cautions Brody. "Nonablative lasers do something to scars, but, so far, they just don't seem to do that much."

Alster, who has done extensive research on laser scar treatment and conducted numerous clinical trials with nonablative lasers, is more enthusiastic about their potential, but warns that treatment with nonablative lasers remains highly unpredictable. "I have seen some really amazing results on acne scars. After a series of five treatments, some patients get as much improvement as I'd expect with CO_2 resurfacing. But others hardly seem to improve at all. The big problem is that right now I can't really tell ahead of time how any one of them will turn out."

FILLERS TO RAISE DEPRESSED SCARS

One of the easiest and least expensive ways to improve the appearance of acne scars is to fill them in with injected or implanted substances that push up the depressions. As well as supplementing resurfacing procedures, fillers can be used on their own, for immediate improvement. They are most effective on soft-sided, distensible scars (those you can stretch out) and in some cases can be used successfully to fill in the small gap left behind following subcision surgery to release broad, bound-down scars. They do not work at all on ice-pick scars. (Material placed beneath an ice-pick acne scar will only elevate the skin around the edges, creating a kind of doughnut effect around the pit.)

The world of cosmetic fillers is a confusing and perpetually changing one, with new substances continuously being introduced, refined, and breathlessly proclaimed in the pages of

women's magazines to be the latest miracle in facial rejuvena-
tion. But beware: Injectable and implanted materials are regulated by the FDA as "medical devices," like artificial hip joints
or heart valves, not drugs. Thus they are not subject to the same
rigorous premarket approval process as prescription medicines.
One group, called allogenic products, which are derived from
human sources such as cadavers, are regarded as transplanted
donor tissue, and are even more leniently regulated.

Also be aware that not all of these substances are suitable for
acne scar correction, cautions San Francisco's Glogau, an authority on cosmetic fillers with years of experience in using
them to repair acne scars. "You have to be very careful that you
don't wind up as a guinea pig for some guy who happens to have
some stuff in his refrigerator that he just assumes will work on
your scars. That happens a lot more often than you'd expect."

INJECTIONS

Generally, fluid filler materials that are injected beneath scars
offer the quickest results on acne scars. Typically, the appearance of the scar improves instantly, although there may be
some downtime to recover from local swelling, redness, or
bruising from the injection itself. Also, doctors may deliber-
ately "overcorrect" some scars, injecting a little additional
material to compensate for shrinkage. Overcorrected scars
may appear somewhat swollen or lumpy for several days
before settling down.

Injected filler material can be divided into two broad categories: biodegradable and permanent. Biodegradable materials
are derived from animal or human tissues. Their drawback is
their impermanence. In most instances the body eventually
absorbs the injected material and the depression returns. It is

difficult to predict how long this will take; the effects of the filler may last anywhere from a few months to a year or more. However, repeated injections over the course of many years can lead to more lasting results.

"I still see some of those patients who were in the original collagen trials back in 1974 and 1975," says Glogau. "For the most part, they had their acne scars treated repeatedly, right through the 1980s. And now they don't need any injections. I think that's because you get a little reaction each time you inject a scar, and eventually the wounding process may lead to a permanent correction."

Synthetic permanent materials can also be a good choice for acne scars, he notes. "In fact, that's exactly how I think permanent fillers should be used—like we used to use liquid silicone in the old days—for small defects, not in large quantities for dynamic expression lines or volume augmentation, which unfortunately is where these substances usually wind up—filling big lines in the forehead or around the mouth." Used in large quantities, he warns, permanent fillers are more likely to produce unwelcome side effects, in particular, what is known as a granulomous response, which results in a permanent hard red lump in the injected spot.

That can, in fact, also happen with the small amounts used for individual acne scars. "This is a really difficult risk to assess. You can inject a hundred acne scars and get a granulomous response in just one. So you need to be cautious." Glogau advises using permanent filler materials slowly and very sparingly. "Just a tiny fraction of a drop, four or five times, over a year and a half, for an acne scar."

Animal-Derived Collagen Injections (*Zyderm, Zyplast, Artefill*)
The oldest product available for scar filling, bovine collagen (derived from cows) remains popular for its predictability and

cost-effectiveness. (The price of injections starts at about $150 apiece.) It is available as Zyderm, the original formula, useful for shallow scars, and Zyplast, a somewhat denser, longer-lasting collagen used to fill deeper depressions. Artefill, a permanent filler, is a combination product—bovine collagen mixed with Plexiglas microbeads that provide a permanent correction after the collagen has been absorbed by the body. Because of the potential for an allergic reaction to animal collagen, two skin-patch tests, two weeks apart, are required six weeks prior to treatment with any of these substances.

Human Collagen Injections (CosmoDerm, CosmoPlast, Autologen)

Because they are much less likely to cause allergic reactions, human collagen injections are becoming an increasingly popular alternative to the standard bovine collagen. CosmoDerm and CosmoPlast are bioengineered human tissue versions of Zyderm and Zyplast; they are derived from human fibroblast cells grown in the laboratory. "These are fine for acne scars," says Dr. Glogau. "In fact, they are interchangeable with Zyderm and Zyplast and will probably replace them." Autologen, derived from your own tissue harvested during cosmetic surgery procedures such as tummy tucks and face-lifts, is a far less practical choice. "This is basically a niche product that appeals to plastic surgeons who are already cutting things up and don't want to throw anything away. But the average acne patient isn't going to want to have surgery just to generate material to correct her scars."

Fascia Injections (Fascian)

Harvested from cadavers, Fascian is preserved connective tissue (fascia) processed into injectable form. "This is *not* useful for acne scars," says Glogau. "And anyone who tries to tell you it is doesn't know any better. It is too chunky. Basically, you can't get it into the dermis, which is where you want filler for an acne scar. Plus, it's a cadaver product. Cadaver products come from tissue banks; they're not regulated, and I think you'd be crazy to use them."

Hyaluronic Acid Fillers (*Restylane, Hylaform Gel, Perlane*)

Hyaluronic acid gel is a laboratory-engineered product that mimics naturally occurring substances in the dermis. It is the most common cosmetic filler used in other parts of the world, and is rapidly gaining in popularity in the United States. It can be easily injected into the dermis, so it can be used to correct acne scars the same way that collagen can, and in some people it lasts longer than collagen. Its major drawback is that it is a transparent material that, if injected too superficially, produces an effect that turns the overlying skin deep blue. Light enters the skin, hits the substance, goes through a refraction, and bounces back to produce the indigo hue. "This means you have to really know what you're doing to use it, and you can't use it at all for severely atrophic acne scars that are very, very thin," says Glogau. "It will raise them up, but they'll be blue." (The color remains for months, until the body absorbs all the material.)

Autologous Fat

This is fat taken from a patient's own body via liposuction, and then frozen, stored, and gradually reinjected into the face in four or five sessions over the course of a year. It is generally not the best material for acne scars, because fat must be injected into fat, so it has to go into the subcutis. "By definition, an acne scar is in the dermis, so dermal fillers are more effective," comments Glogau. "But you can still get some good results with fat in patients who have very soft atrophic scars that have become more obvious-looking as they age and their skin sags. If you do an all-over volume correction, putting fat back into the face as a whole, it stretches the skin and the scars do look better."

IMPLANTS

Implanted cosmetic filler materials are typically used to fill in large depressed areas, for example, deep facial furrows. They are used on acne scars only in limited instances—for example, in areas where the skin is stiff, such as on the nose or high on the cheekbone, or beneath very broad or linear scars.

Autologous Dermal Grafts

A technique called autologous dermal pocket grafting is sometimes used to correct deep or linear acne scars. A strip of skin is taken from another body location; the epidermis is removed, leaving a sliver of dermal tissue that can be slid, through a small incision, into a pocket tunneled beneath the scar. This typically results in a permanent improvement.

Cadaver Tissue Implants (AlloDerm, Cymetra)

AlloDerm and Cymetra are two trade names for commercially available, freeze-dried dermis, harvested like a donor organ from a body at the time of death. Originally developed as a skin substitute for burn victims, it can be used like an autologous dermal graft, minus the cost and inconvenience of harvesting it from the patient. But, warns Glogau, "It's from cadavers. And these days you've got to worry about where these things come from. I don't recommend it all for cosmetic use."

Synthetic Implants *(GORE S.A.M., Softform)*
Polymer implants have been used in general surgery for twenty years for procedures such as hernia and abdominal wall repairs. The cosmetic versions come in small sheets or hollow polymer tubes, like a child's juice-drink straw, which are implanted beneath deep wrinkles or furrows. Although generally not suitable for acne scars, some surgeons implant little chips of these substances under larger scars.

FINDING A SCAR SPECIALIST

Alster, Brody, Glogau, and Yarborough—all considered by other dermatologists to be among the most skilled and knowledgeable skin surgeons in the world—each has a slightly different set of approaches to acne scarring. But all of them offer exactly the same emphatic advice when it comes to finding a doctor to fix your acne scars: Go all out to find the best-qualified, most experienced scar specialist you can. Take your time. Don't bargain hunt. And although it's important and useful to understand all of the various options when considering acne scar surgery, find the best dermatologic surgeon and let him or her decide about how best to proceed in your case. Repairing acne scars is extremely difficult, and an underqualified practitioner can produce crushingly disappointing results; you'll spend a lot of money and see little or no improvement at all. Or, in the disastrous, worst-case instance, a doctor can actually injure your skin and give you even more terrible scars.

As when selecting any doctor, you can start by asking your own and other physicians to recommend a specialist. You should also contact the American Society for Dermatologic

Surgery at 930 North Meacham Road, Schaumburg, Ill. 60173, or online at www.aboutskinsurgery.com for referrals to surgeons in your area.

Try to come up with the names of at least three doctors to interview, and then make appointments for a consultation with each one. Here are some questions you can take along:

1. "What is your approach to scar revision?"

   Remember, there is no one approach. "If somebody claims they have the latest filler or the latest laser that remodels acne scars, and that is the one thing that person has to offer, then you will know that they are not the best person to treat your scars," warns Brody. "You have to have someone who is experienced in all the different methods, and is equipped to handle all the different types of scars."

2. "How many patients have you treated for acne scarring?"

   You want to be reassured that the doctor has ample experience in a number of different scar revision procedures and is comfortable with all of them.

3. "Can I see before and after photographs of patients you have treated?"

   Physicians with extensive experience should be able to show you photographic samples of their work. Make sure you are seeing pictures of that doctor's own patients. Some doctors use photos obtained from other physicians or from drug or medical equipment companies.

4. "Have you ever published any articles about skin surgery in peer-reviewed journals? Have you ever lectured on the subject to other doctors?"

Notes Alster: "For something as difficult and potentially risky as acne scar repair, you want to find the most experienced and well-regarded · practitioner possible. And really, the very best people tend to be the ones who actively teach or share their experiences with colleagues through publishing or lecturing."

5. "May I talk to some of your patients who have had the same procedure?"

Although most doctors make it a policy not to give out the names of patients under any circumstance, some will put you in touch with those who have volunteered to give a reference. It's worth asking.

Chapter Fourteen

Healing the Inner Scars

As FORMIDABLE A FEAT AS IT IS to repair the physical scars of acne, dealing with the emotional wounds it inflicts can present an even more confounding challenge.

For many people, distress about acne represents what psychotherapists call a "situational" disorder. They are depressed or disheartened by their situation, but when it's gone, when their skin is clear, they're fine. It's as if it never happened.

But others find it hard to get off the emotional hook. Once acne has become part of anyone's identity, it can be difficult to shake off the feelings of unhappiness, self-consciousness, and unworthiness the condition so often engenders. In one study of 193 adults who once had severe acne, yet were now blessed with clear skin, 42 percent of the subjects were not only still extremely insecure about their appearance, they were also more dissatisfied with their lives as a whole than those who had had minimal or moderate acne.

In fact, it is surprisingly common for people who have once had acne to believe they still have it, even after their skin is clear. Yardley, Pennsylvania, dermatologist and psychodermatology expert Richard Fried calls this phenomenon "phantom acne," and likens it to the "phantom fat" that afflicts formerly obese people who still feel they are overweight even after they have lost their excess poundage.

Even if you have a more realistic view of your own skin, you may experience similar feelings. After years of thinking there is something wrong with the way you look, you may automatically come to believe there is something wrong with yourself—no matter what the state of your skin. These negative feelings become habits—whether they are reinforced by the presence of active breakouts and visible scars, or bolstered by unhappy memories.

But you can break these habits. One way is to employ some of the empowering, control-enhancing tools outlined on pages 143–145: engaging in exercise, embracing formal stress-reduction techniques, proactively caring for your skin, learning about acne so that you don't get caught in the trap of perceiving it as a personal failure, and seeking professional therapy if needed.

And you can take other steps to reclaim parts of your life that acne may have stolen. "What I see from so many acne patients is a real withdrawal from life," says Fried. "They put off living the life they want. They say, 'I'm going to join that club . . .' 'I'm going to take that class . . .' 'I'm going to go after that job . . . *when my acne clears up.*' Well, part of the process of breaking free from acne has got to be deciding to get out and live regardless of how much acne you have, or how bad the scars are, or how traumatic your memories are. Because if you don't, you've become a cripple."

Acne is particularly insidious in the way it robs you of activity, so start by taking an honest inventory of the things you avoid. Fried suggests sitting down and literally making a list. Do you sometimes avoid social events? Do you shy away from certain situations because you know you are going to have to meet people or stand up in front of them? What about sports or hobbies? Do you avoid the golf course or the ski slopes because the light is too harsh? Do you never swim or play tennis because your makeup will come off? In fact, while you're at it, ask yourself how much time you spend touching up your face, or checking your reflection in mirrors or store windows. Ask yourself what you used to do for fun, and what you would really like to do now.

Next, start looking for ways to reclaim those positive aspects of your life. "You know, the old view of psychotherapy used to be, 'Let's get them on the couch, and when we've explored enough issues and acquired enough insight, then we'll tell the patients they can go out and function,'" says Fried. "Well, we've learned that you get much better results with patients by telling them to just go do something. Go for a walk, play a game, go to a movie, go to a party. Every study shows that the more you can encourage people to function, the better they will do. It's the 'as if' school of therapy. If you behave 'as if' you are healthy and happy long enough, the emotions will follow."

Then take the final, hardest step: Really look at your acne, fully acknowledge how much influence it has had on your life, and make a conscious decision not to let it continue to do that. Don't try to distract yourself from it or pretend it doesn't exist, but in a relaxed, focused, and controlled fashion, face whatever pain is there and make a choice as to how much you are going to let it interfere with your life from now on.

It occurs to me as I write these words that they may sound impossibly Pollyanna-like, even a little loopy in their insistence on talking yourself into feeling better. But the fact is, if you feel bad about yourself or limited in any way because of acne, you simply cannot escape those feelings by trying to ignore or evade them.

"So often what we want to do when we see something we perceive as painful or unsightly is to turn our head away from it as quickly as we can," says Fried. "And I think that using meditation or self-thought techniques can help with this. Say, 'I do have acne; I do have acne scars. I don't like it. I understand that other people may react to it. But it is what it is, and I don't want to react in such a strong negative fashion. I don't want it to own as much of my time and emotions as it does. And now I won't let it.'"

I did not receive that particular piece of advice myself until I had almost finished writing this book. Up until then, I had never consciously applied any particularly heartfelt appraisal, or determination to change, to my own feelings about my skin. Not consciously. However, through the sheer luck of having the opportunity to write about acne, I fell into a situation in which confronting negative feelings about it occurred as a matter of course.

When I began to learn about other women's acne—and to talk about it and deal with it—I found myself embracing the very subject I had tried to avoid for most of my life. After years of running and hiding from acne, but never escaping it, I was suddenly looking it in the face every day. And it lost its power.

Today, for the first time ever, I feel really free—strangely, even miraculously, unaffected by the state of my own skin.

I hope that reading this will help you as well, and that you will find your way not just to clear skin but to a clear heart.

Appendix A

----◦----

Acne Drugs in Pregnancy

It is, of course, critical for every pregnant woman or nursing mother to thoroughly discuss *every* medicine she takes (including over-the-counter and herbal or other alternative remedies) with her obstetrician/gynecologist and any other specialist who has prescribed or recommended medicines to her. Acne drugs are no exception; even medicines applied to the skin can be absorbed into the system and may affect a developing fetus or breast-fed baby.

Prescription Drugs

Since 1979, the U.S. Food and Drug Administration has divided prescription drugs into five "Use-in-Pregnancy" categories, A, B, C, D, and X. (The same rating applies to both oral and topical forms of the drug.) The rankings essentially weigh the degree to which human or animal studies have demonstrated the risk of any given drug to a developing fetus, against the potential benefits of that drug to a patient.

Category A: Controlled studies show no risk. Studies in pregnant women have failed to show a risk to the fetus in any trimester. (None of the common prescription acne medicines fall into this category.)

Category B: No evidence of risk in humans. Studies in pregnant women have not shown any risk of fetal abnormality in humans, but animal studies have demonstrated increased risk; or there have been no studies of pregnant women, although animal studies show no risk. The risk appears remote, although possible.

Category B acne drugs include: azelaic acid (Azelex, Finevin); erythromycin, oral (Ery-Tab and others) and topical (Emgel and others); clindamycin, oral and topical (Cleocin, Clinac, Cindagel, Clindets, and others); metronidazole (MetroGel, MetroCream, MetroLotion, Noritate).

Category C: Risk cannot be ruled out. There have been no human or animal studies that rule out risk. Or animal studies have shown a risk. There is a chance of fetal harm; however, the potential benefits to the patient may outweigh the risks. Should only be used by a pregnant woman if clearly needed. (Because acne is not a severe medical condition, many doctors do not recommend category C acne drugs in pregnancy.)

Category C acne drugs include: adapalene (Differin); benzoyl peroxide (Brevoxyl, Triaz); antibiotic–benzoyl peroxide combinations (BenzaClin, Benzamycin); sodium sulfacetimide (Klaron, Sulfacet, and others); tretinoin (Retin-A, Renova, Avita).

Also: Dapsone, spironolactone (Aldactone, Alatone), and oral corticosteroids (Prednisone, Dexamethasone), which may be prescribed to treat acne.

Category D: Positive evidence of risk. Controlled studies in humans or statistical evidence have demonstrated fetal risk. Drugs in this category would not be used in pregnancy except in rare circumstances—for example, if the mother were suffering from a life-threatening condition for which no safer alternative was available.

Category D acne drugs include: doxycycline (Adoxa, Doryx, Monodox, Vibramycin); minocycline (Dynacin; Minocin); tetracycline.

Also: flutamide (Euflex, Euflexin), which may be prescribed to treat acne.

Category X: Contraindicated in pregnancy. Human and animal studies, or reports from users of the drug, have positively demonstrated that the drug causes fetal abnormalities; the risk outweighs any benefit to the patient.

Category X acne drugs include: isotretinoin (Accutane, Amnesteem, Claravis, Sotret); tazarotene (Tazorac, Avage).

Also: Hormonal therapies that may be used to treat acne, such as birth control pills (for example, Alesse, Estrostep, Ortho Tri-Cyclen, Yasmin, Diane, Dianette), or finasteride (Propecia, Proscar).

OVER-THE-COUNTER AND ALTERNATIVE THERAPIES

Unlike prescription medications, over-the-counter acne treatments are not categorized for pregnancy risk. Still, even if you deem them to be safe, it is wise to clear any OTC acne product with your doctor.

The effects of herbs and dietary supplements are even more problematic; experts say don't assume that if a product is labeled "natural," it is safe for a developing fetus. So check with your doctor.

For further information about drugs and pregnancy, you can contact the Organization of Teratology and Information Services (888-285-3410; online at www.otispregnancy.org) or the Canadian site for pregnancy safety issues, www.motherisk.org. The *PDR for Herbal Medicines* and *PDR for Nutritional Supplements*, both available at public libraries, also contain information about the known risks of herbal and nutritional therapies.

Appendix B

---◆◇◆---

Resources

A rapidly increasing number of new, over-the-counter acne products, along with the advent of Internet shopping, has put an unprecedented number of excellent, affordable, nonprescription acne products within reach of virtually everyone. The lists that follow are a very small sample; they are assembled principally to serve as examples of key nonprescription treatments discussed in the preceding pages.

For the most part, they are drawn from the most common and familiar acne lines (for example, Clean & Clear, Clearasil, Neutrogena, Oxy, Phisoderm). These are all widely available in mass retail outlets; they can also be ordered online at www.drugstore.com. Other included acne products—DDF, Joey, Peter Thomas Roth, and Murad Acne—are available at specialty stores or online at www.beauty.com.

Proactiv, the best-selling U.S. acne brand, is available at www.proactiv.com, or by phoning 800-950-4695.

Clinique, the best-selling department store acne treatment brand, can also be found online at www.clinique.com.

Paula's Choice, a well-priced, no-frills line developed by consumer writer Paula Begoun, is available at www.cosmticcop.com, or by phoning 800-831-4088.

Cleansers

Appropriate cleansers for acne-prone skin can be divided into two broad categories: nonmedicated and medicated. Because many acne treatment products (both prescription and nonprescription) are intrinsically drying and/or irritating, dermatologists often recommend cleansing only with gentle, nonmedicated bar or liquid products, such as the examples below. These are also generally preferred for women with mature skin that tends to be dry, sensitive, or prone to rosacea; or for anyone starting a topical retinoid or taking Accutane.

Bar Cleansers

Acne-Aid Cleansing Bar for Deep Pore Cleansing	Neutrogena Transparent Facial Bar
Basis Sensitive Skin Bar	Oil of Olay Beauty Bar
Dove Beauty Bar	Purpose Gentle Cleaning Bar

Lotion or Liquid Cleansers

Aquanil Lotion	Eucerin Pore Purifying Foaming Wash
Basis Liquid Cleanser	Neutrogena Extra Gentle Cleanser
Cetaphil Facial Cleanser for Normal to Oily Skin	Neutrogena Foaming Face Wash
Cetaphil Gentle Skin Cleanser	Paula's Choice One Step Cleanser
Eucerin Gentle Hydrating Cleanser	Purpose Liquid Cleanser

MEDICATED ACNE CLEANSERS

Medicated acne cleansers typically contain either benzoyl peroxide or salicylic acid. Because they are rinsed off the skin, they tend to be less effective than leave-on benzoyl peroxide or salicylic acid treatments, but they can be helpful as adjuncts to those products or as an alternative for anyone with sensitive skin. They may also serve as a means to condition skin for stronger, leave-on products.

Benzoyl Peroxide Cleansers

These act to reduce follicle-dwelling, inflammation-provoking *P. acnes* bacteria. (Note that many antibacterial cleansers marketed for blemished or "problem" skin contain the active ingredient triclosan, which is not an acne medication and is not considered to be effective against *P. acnes* in sebaceous follicles. Don't confuse these with acne cleansers containing benzoyl peroxide.)

Clean & Clear Continuous Control Daily Cleanser (10%)	Peter Thomas Roth Medicated BPO 10% Acne Wash
DDF Medicated Skin Cleanser (5%)	Peter Thomas Roth Medicated BPO 5% Acne Wash
DDF Pumice Acne Scrub (2.5%)	Proactiv Renewing Cleanser (2.5%)
Neutrogena Clear Pore Cleanser/Mask (3.5%)	ZAPZYT Treatment Bar, 10% Benzoyl Peroxide
Oxy 10 Balance Oil-Free Maximum Strength Acne Wash (10%)	

Salicylic Acid Cleansers

Salicylic acid cleansers are designed to exfoliate the skin's surface and reduce comedones in the follicles. They work most effectively at concentrations of 2 percent, in an acid base, with a pH under 4; so if you are relying on one of these cleansers to work as your principal exfoliant or comedolytic treatment, choose one with a 2 percent concentration and a low pH, and plan to leave the lather on for at least sixty seconds so your skin can absorb the active ingredient before you rinse.

(The pH values given in the right-hand column of the following chart, and in the two salicylic acid treatment product charts on pages 211–212, are the result of my tests with a school laboratory digital pH meter. If you are curious about the pH of other products, you can use inexpensive pH testing papers, available at laboratory supply outlets, such as Micro Essential Laboratory Inc. in Brooklyn, New York, at www.microessentialslab.com, or by phone at 718-338-3618.)

Aveeno Clear Complexion Foaming Cleanser	.5%	4.81
Bioré Blemish Fighting Cleanser	.5%	6.96
Clean & Clear Continuous Control Acne Wash, Oil Free	2%	4.72
Clearasil 3 in 1 Acne Defense Cleanser	2%	3.07
Clearasil Total Control Deep Pore Cream Cleanser	2%	3.05
Clearasil Icewash Acne Gel Cleanser	2%	3.6
Clinique Acne Solutions Cleansing Foam	1%	5.75
DDF Therapeutic Skincare, Salicylic Wash 2%	2%	4.9
L'Oreal Pure Zone Pore Unclogging Scrub Cleanser	1%	5.05
L'Oreal Pure Zone Skin Balancing Cream Cleanser	2%	4.5
Murad Acne Clarifying Cleanser	1.5%	4.1
Neutrogena Healthy Skin Anti-Wrinkle Anti-Blemish Cleanser	.5%	4.10
Neutrogena Oil-Free Acne Wash	2%	4.13
Neutrogena Oil-Free Acne Wash Foam Cleanser	2%	4.03
Neutrogena Oil Free Cream Cleanser	2%	4.0
Peter Thomas Roth Beta Hydroxy Acid 2% Acne Wash	2%	4.18
PHisoderm Clear Confidence Facial Wash	2%	4.64
ZAPZYT Acne Wash Treatment	2 %	3.97

BENZOYL PEROXIDE TREATMENTS

Benzoyl peroxide lotions, creams, or gels, which act principally by killing inflammation-causing *P. acnes* bacteria, are the most potent acne-fighting treatment products you can get without a prescription. Although often marketed as spot treatments, they work best as preventive medicine, applied consistently to all acne-prone areas of skin at least once a day. Higher-percentage benzoyl peroxide products offer only minimal gains in effectiveness, but are far more irritating, so try to stick to a 2.5 percent concentration, 5 percent at most. (You may need the higher concentration if your skin is very oily.) The 10 percent products are best suited for excessively oily teenage skin.

Benzoyl Peroxide 2.5%

Klear Action (sold as a set with a 2.5% BP cleanser and a glycolic acid toner in "Klear Action Acne Treatment System")	Peter Thomas Roth BPO Gel 2.5%
Neutrogena On-the-Spot Acne Treatment Vanishing Formula	Proactiv Repairing Lotion (available separately, or with a BP cleanser and a glycolic acid toner in Proactiv Solution's "3-piece system")
Paula's Choice Blemish Fighting Solution, All Skin Types	Stridex Day & Night Acne Medication (part of 2-part set, sold with a 2% salicylic acid lotion)

Benzoyl Peroxide 5%

Clearasil Vanishing Acne Treatment Overnight Acne Defense Gel	Oxy Balance Acne Treatment for Sensitive Skin, Vanishing Formula
Clinique Acne Solutions Emergency Gel Lotion	Paula's Choice Extra Strength Blemish Fighting Solution
DDF Benzoyl Peroxide Gel 5% with Tea Tree Oil	Peter Thomas Roth BPO Gel 5%
Nature's Cure (sold as part of homeopathic "Two-Part Acne Treatment System for Females")	Proactiv Advanced Blemish Treatment

Benzoyl Peroxide 10%

Clean & Clear Persa-Gel 10 Maximum Strength	Oxy Balance Maximum Acne Treatment, Vanishing
Clearasil Maximum Strength Acne Treatment Cream, Tinted	Peter Thomas Roth BPO Gel 10%
Clearasil Maximum Strength Acne Treatment Cream, Vanishing	ZAPZYT 10% Benzoyl Peroxide

SALICYLIC ACID TREATMENTS

Salicylic acid treatment products work to reduce inflammation, exfoliate the skin surface, expel small comedones, and prevent new ones from forming. But remember, salicylic acid is most effective as an exfoliant/comedolytic at the highest (2 percent) concentration and in an acid base (with a pH of less than 4); it diminishes in effectiveness as the concentration goes down and the pH increases beyond 4. However, low-concentration, higher pH products tend to be gentler on the skin and will still work to counter inflammation. Also, increasingly, salicylic acid acne products (in particular those aimed at the adult market) are likely to contain additional anti-inflammatory components such as vitamins, minerals, antioxidants, botanical and herbal ingredients that may act to boost their inflammation-fighting qualities.

.5%–1% Salicylic Acid Treatments

Aveeno Clear Complexion Astringent	.5%	4.01
Aveeno Clear Complexion Daily Moisturizer	.5%	3.76
Clean & Clear Blackhead Clearing Astringent	1%	2.9
Clean & Clear Clarifying Toner	.5%	3.97
Clean & Clear Deep Cleaning Astringent, Sensitive Skin	.5%	4.21
Clean & Clear Oil Free Dual Action Moisturizer	.5%	4.10
Clearasil Total Control Daily Skin Perfecting Treatment	.5%	4.61
Joey New York Chin Breakout Relief	1 %	6.00
Joey New York Pure Pores Blackhead Remover and Pore Minimizer Gel	.5%	3.83
Joey New York Pure Pores Roll-On Blemish Fix	1%	2.58
L'Oreal Pure Zone Skin Relief Oil-Free Moisturizer	.6%	6.40
Neutrogena Blackhead Eliminating Astringent	.5%	3.81
Neutrogena Blackhead Eliminating Treatment Mask	.5%	4.17
Neutrogena Multi-Vitamin Acne Treatment Lotion	1.5%	3.8
Murad Acne Moisturizing Acne Treatment Gel	.5%	5.07
Murad Acne Exfoliating Acne Treatment Gel	1 %	3.7
Paula's Choice 1% Beta Hydroxy Liquid Solution, Normal to Oily Skin	1%	3.15

2% Salicylic Acid Treatments

Clean & Clear Deep Cleaning Astringent	2.6
Clean & Clear Invisible Blemish Treatment	3.67
Clearasil Acne Fighting Facial Moisturizer, Dual Action	3.07
Clearasil Overnight Acne Defense Gel	3.38
Clearasil Pore Cleansing Astringent	3.63
Clinique Night Treatment Gel	3.82
L'Oreal Pure Zone Pore Tightening Astringent	3.82
L'Oreal Pure Zone Spot Check Blemish Treatment	4.13
Neutrogena Body Clear Lotion, Salicylic Acid Acne Treatment	4.11
Neutrogena Clear Pore Oil-Controlling Astringent	2.69
Neutrogena Clear Pore Soothing Gel Astringent	4.63
Neutrogena Rapid Clear Acne Eliminating Gel	4.44
Neutrogena Nighttime Pore Clarifying Gel	4.47
Paula's Choice 2% Beta Hydroxy Liquid Solution, All Skin Types	3.98
Philosophy Hope in a Bottle, Topical Treatment for Adult Acne	3.6
Philosophy On a Clear Day, Blemish Gel for Adult Acne	3.34
PHisoderm Clear Confidence Blemish Masque	7.75
PHisoderm Clear Confidence Clear Swab	4.73
Stridex Day & Night Acne Medication (part of 2-part set, sold with a 2.5% BP lotion)	4.72
ZAPZYT Pore Treatment Gel	3.48

ADDITIONAL ACNE TREATMENT PRODUCTS

Glycolic Acid

Unlike salicylic acid, glycolic acid is not oil soluble, so it does not penetrate sebaceous follicles to loosen comedones or prevent them from forming. However, toners and gels containing glycolic acid (AHA) may be incorporated into an acne-fighting regimen to exfoliate the skin surface and remove external debris that can clog pores and worsen acne.

DDF Glycolic Gel 10%	Peter Thomas Roth Glycolic Acid 10% Clarifying Gel
Proactiv Revitalizing Toner	Peter Thomas Roth Glycolic Acid Clarifying Tonic

Sulfur

Although relatively rare these days, acne products containing sulfur can be useful as spot treatments, concealers, or treatment masks to get the red out of active acne. Acnomel, Liquimat, and Rezamid are traditional acne products that can still be found at some drugstores (or pharmacists can order them for you); they are also available though the Internet. Try www.medichest.com for Acnomel and www.dermstore.com for Liquimat and Rezamid.

Acnomel (8% sulfur; 2% resorcinol)	Peter Thomas Roth Therapeutic Sulfur Masque Acne Treatment (10% sulfur)
Clearasil Adult Care Acne Treatment Cream (8% sulfur; 2% resorcinol)	Proactiv Solution Concealer Plus (8% sulfur)
Liquimat Acne Treatment and Cover-up Lotion (4% sulfur)	Proactiv Solution Refining Mask (6% sulfur)
Murad Acne Clarifying Mask (4% sulfur)	Rezamid Acne Treatment Lotion (5% sulfur; 2% resorcinol)
Murad Acne Spot Treatment (3% sulfur)	

Oil-Absorbing Products

Many acne treatment lines and cosmetic companies offer some kind of oil-absorbing skin preparation (or "mattifier") to be worn alone or under makeup to reduce shine. If your skin is exceptionally oily, however, your best bet is one of the patented oil-control products: Seban or (even more effective, although slightly more expensive) Clinac OC Oil Control Gel, derived from technology used to mop up oil spills in the ocean. Both are available at pharmacies, or by mail order. You can order Seban at www.cooperlabs.com or by phone at 800-645-5048. Order Clinac OC at either www.dermstore.com or www.dermdoctor.com.

BIBLIOGRAPHY

ABBREVIATIONS

AAD American Academy of Dermatology
Arch Derm *Archives of Dermatology*
Br J Derm *British Journal of Dermatology*
Derm Clinics *Dermatologic Clinics*
Derm Times *Dermatology Times*
JAAD *Journal of the American Academy of Dermatology*
JAMA *Journal of the American Medical Association*
NEJM *New England Journal of Medicine*
S&A *Skin and Aging*
S&A News *Skin and Allergy News*

General References

Bergfeld, Wilma F., and Richard B. Odom, eds. "New Perspectives on Acne." *Clinician* 12.2 (1994): 4–30.

Cunliffe, William J., and Harald P. M. Gollnick. *Acne: Diagnosis and Management*. London: Martin Dunitz, 2001.

Fulton, James E. *Acne RX*. James E. Fulton, Jr., 2001.

Gollnick, Harald P. M., and William J. Cunliffe, eds. "Management of Acne: A Report from a Global Alliance to Improve Outcomes in Acne." *JAAD* 49.1 (2003): S1–37.

Lehmann, Harold P., John S. Andrews, et al. "Management of Acne: Volume 1: Evidence Report and Appendixes." Agency for Healthcare Research and Quality, Department of Health and Human Services. AHRQ Publication No. 01-E019. September 2001.

Parker, James N., and Philip M. Parker. *The 2002 Patients' Sourcebook on Acne*. San Diego: Icon Group International, Inc., 2002.

Plewig, Gerd, and Albert M. Kligman. *Acne and Rosacea*. 3d edition. Berlin, Heidelberg, New York: Springer-Verlag, 2000.

Chapter 1: Facing Up to Acne

Barnes, Julian E. "A New Age in Acne Treatment: It's No Longer Just a Market for Teenagers." *The New York Times.* 27 April 2001.

Gouldon, V., S. M. Clark, and W. J. Cunliffe. "Post-Adolescent Acne: A Review of Clinical Features." *Br J Derm* 136.1 (1997): 66–70.

Shaw, James C., and L. White. "Persistent Acne in Adult Women." *Arch Derm.* 137.9 (2001): 1252–53.

Stern, R. S. "The Prevalence of Acne on the Basis of Physical Examination." *JAAD* 26.6 (1992): 931–35.

TalkSurgery. "Chronic Acne—No Longer Just a Teenage Concern." Available from http.//www.talksurgery.com/consumer/new/new000001_1.htl.

Chapter 2: Breaking Free

Crissey, John T., Lawrence C. Parrish, and Karl Holubar. *Historical Atlas of Dermatology and Dermatologists.* New York: Parthenon Publishing Group, 2002.

Cunliffe, William J., and J. A. Cotterill. *The Acnes: Clinical Features, Pathogenesis and Management.* London: W. B. Saunders Company, 1975.

Drake, Lynn A. "Psychosocial Effects of Acne and Rosacea." *Perspectives: Current Concepts in Acne and Rosacea.* Symposium at the American Academy of Dermatology, Orlando, Fla., July 1996.

Jelinek, John E. "Acne: 10 Common Myths—and the Facts." *Consultant* (May 1979).

Lasek, R. J., and M. Chren. "Acne Vulgaris and the Quality of Life of Adult Dermatology Patients." *Arch Derm* 134 (1998): 454–58.

Lookingbill, Donald. "Psychologic Manifestation and the Emotional Impact of Acne." *Acne Briefs* 1.6 (1999). Available from http.//www.academymedpublish.com/Acne_Briefs/ACNEv1n6.txt.

Chapter 3: Understanding Acne

Ingham, Eileen. "Inflammation in Acne Vulgaris." Available from http.//www.leeds.ac.uk/src/srcimm1.html.

Leyden, James J. "New Understandings of the Pathogenesis of Acne." *JAAD* 32 (1995): S15–25.

Oberemok, Steve S., and Alan R. Shalita. "Acne Vulgaris I: Pathogenesis and Diagnosis." *Cutis* 70.2 (2002): 101–5

Taylor, Susan C., ed. "Understanding Skin of Color." *JAAD* 46.2 (2003): S41–62, S98–106.

Webster, Guy. "Acne Vulgaris: State of the Science." *Arch Derm* 135 (1999): 1101–02.

White, Gary M. "Recent Findings in the Epidemiologic Evidence, Classification, and Subtypes of Acne Vulgaris." *JAAD* 39.2 (1998): S34–37.

Chapter 4: "Will It Make Me Break Out?"

Baumann, Leslie. "Cosmeceutical Critique: DHEA." *S&A News* 32.12 (2001): 33.

Canadian Center for Occupational Health and Safety. "OSH Answers: Diseases, Disorders & Injuries. Acne." Available from http://www.ccohs.ca/oshanswers/diseases/acne.html.

Connolly, C. S., and J. Bikowski. "As Summer Continues, Remember the Role of Heat and Friction in Acne." *S&A* 9.8 (2001).

Draelos, Zoe Diana. "Cosmetic Conundrums: Why Do Some Cosmetics and Skincare Products Cause Breakouts?" *Derm Times* (May 2002).

Kuznar, Wayne. "Acne Sufferers Need Not Avoid Oily Cosmetics." *Derm Times* (Supplement, September 1997): S27.

Larkin, Marilyn. "DHEA: Will Science Confirm the Headlines?" *Lancet* 352.9123 (1998).

Lebwohl, Mark. "Acne and Rosacea Clinical Pearls." Presented at AAD annual meeting, Washington, D.C., 4 March 2001.

Scheman, Andrew. "Adverse Reaction to Cosmetics." *Derm Clinics* 18.4 (2000): 685–96.

Simion, F. Anthony. "Acnegenicity and Comedogenicity Testing for Cosmetics." In *Handbook of Cosmetic Science and Technology*, edited by Andre O. Barel, Marc Payer, and Howard I. Maibach. New York, Basel: Marcel Dekker, 2001: 837–44.

Chapter 5: Over-the-Counter Remedies

Begoun, Paula. *The Beauty Bible*. 2d edition. Seattle: Beginning Press, 2002.

Dubrow, Terry J., and Brenda A. Adderly. *The Acne Cure*. Rodale Press, 2003.

Baumann, Leslie. "Cosmeceuticals: Drugs versus Cosmetics" and "Moisturizing Agents." In *Cosmetic Dermatology: Principles and Practice*. New York: McGraw-Hill, 2002: 197–98, 93–97.

Ertel, Keith. "Modern Skin Cleansers." *Derm Clinics* 15.4 (2002): 561–75.

Food and Drug Administration. Code of Federal Regulations, Title 21, Volume 5, Part 333—Topical Antimicrobial Drug Products for Over-the-Counter Human Use—Table; Subpart D—Topical Acne Drug Products. Sec. 333-310 Acne Active Ingredients [Revised as of April 1, 2001].

Fulghum D. D., et al. "Abrasive Cleansing in the Management of Acne Vulgaris." *Arch Derm* 118.9 (1982).

Kligman, Albert M. "Cosmetics: A Dermatologist Looks to the Future: Promises and Problems." *Derm Clinics* 18.4 (2000): 699–709.

Kligman, Douglas. "Cosmeceuticals." *Derm Clinics* 18.4 (2000): 609–15.

Lamberg, Lynne. "Treatment Cosmetics: Hype or Help?" *JAMA*. Available from http://jama.ama-ssn.org/issues/v279n20/full/jmn0527-1.html.

Lee, Lisa. "Clear, Healthy Skin Today." *Self* (October 2002): 201.

Leyden, James J., et al. "A Double-Blind Placebo Controlled Evaluation of a Stabilized Retinol/Salicylic Acid Treatment on Acne-Prone Aged Facial Skin." Poster at AAD annual meeting, New Orleans, La., 26 February 2002.

Murphy, Robert. "Cosmeceuticals: Can the Science Support the Claims?" *S&A* 9.3 (2001).

Chapter 6: Prescription Treatment

Bershad, Susan. "The Modern Age of Acne Therapy: A Review of Current Treatment Options." *Mt. Sinai Journal of Medicine* 68.4-5 (2001): 279–86.

——. "Topical Retinoids: Alternative Dosing Strategies." Presented at AAD annual meeting, New Orleans, La., 26 February 2002.

Coates, P., S. Vyakrman, E. A. Eady, et al. "Prevalence of Antibiotic-Resistant Propionibacteria on the Skin of Acne Patients: 10-Year Surveillance Data and Snapshot Distribution Study." *Br J Derm* 146.5 (2002): 840.

Cunliffe, William J. "New Insights into P. Acnes Resistance." Presented at AAD annual meeting, Washington, D.C., 4 March 2001.

Del Rosso, James Q. "Retinoic Acid Receptors and Topical Acne Therapy: Establishing the Link Between Gene Expression and Drug Efficacy." *Cutis* 70.2 (2002): 127–29.

Dermatology Prescribing Guide. Montvale, N.J.: Medical Economics, 2002.

Graupe, K., W. Cunliffe, H. Gollnick, et al. "Efficacy and Safety of Topical Azelaic Acid (20% Cream): An Overview of Results from European Clinical Trials and Experimental Reports." *Cutis* 57 (1996): 13–9.

Grimes, Pearl E. "Using Tazarotene to Treat Acne in Patients with Skin Type V or VI." Poster at AAD annual meeting, San Francisco, Calif., March 2000.

————. "Acne in Darker Racial Ethnic Groups: Special Considerations." *Update of Topical Retinoid Therapy.* Highlights from a symposium held during the 25th Hawaii Dermatology Seminar, 7 February 2001.

————. "Acne: Special Issues in Treatment of Darker Skin Types." Presented at AAD annual meeting, San Francisco, Calif., 11 March 2000.

Guttman, Cheryl. "Cosmeceutical Adjuncts May Circumvent Tretinoin Effects." *Derm Times* (1 February 2002).

————. "Issues Influence Antimicrobial Treatment Decisions." *Derm Times* (1 September 2002).

Halder, Rebat M. "The Role of Retinoids in the Management of Cutaneous Conditions in Blacks." *JAAD* 39.2 (1998): S98–103.

Jancin, Bruce. "Blacks Prone to Severe Minocycline Reaction." *S&A News* 29.4 (1997): 33.

Kligman, A. "The Growing Importance of Topical Retinoids in Clinical Dermatology: A Retrospective and Prospective Analysis." *JAAD* 39. 2 (1998): S2–7.

————. "The Treatment of Acne with Topical Retinoids: One Man's Opinions." *JAAD* 36.6 (1997): 592–95.

Knowles, Sandra R., L. Shapiro, and N. H. Sher. "Serious Adverse Reactions Induced by Minocycline." *Arch Derm* 132 (1996): 934–38.

Leyden, James J., ed. "Improving Acne Outcomes with Combination Therapy." *JAAD* 49.3 (2003): S199–232.

————. "Topical Retinoids: First Line for Inflammatory Acne?" Presented at AAD annual meeting, New Orleans, La., 26 February 2002.

————. "Topical Retinoids: New Insights." Presented at AAD annual meeting, Washington, D.C., 4 March 2001.

Lookingbill, Donald P., D. K. Chalker, J. S. Lindholm, et al. "Treatment of Acne with a Combination Clindamycin/Benzoyl Peroxide Gel, Benzoyl Peroxide Gel and Vehicle Gel: Combined Results of Two Double-Blind Investigations." *JAAD* 37 (1997): 590–95.

Lucky, Anne, S. Cullen, T. Funicella, et al. "Double-Blind, Vehicle-Controlled, Multi-Center Comparison of Two 0.02% Tretinoin Creams in Patients with Acne Vulgaris." *JAAD* 38 (1998): 524–30.

Mechcatie, Elizabeth. "Blue Light Special for Moderate Acne." *S&A News* 33.10 (2002): 1.

Milliken, L. "Acne Briefs." Vol. 3, no. 5, 2001. Available from http://www.academymedpublish.com/Acne_Briefs/ACNEv3n5.txt.

Oberemok, Steve S., and A. R. Shalita, "Acne Vulgaris II: Treatment." *Cutis* 70.2 (2002): 111–14.

Shalita, A.R., J. S. Weiss, D. K. Chalker, et al. "A Comparison of the Efficacy and Safety of Adapalene Gel 0.1% and Tretinoin Gel 0.025% in the Treatment of Acne Vulgaris: A Multicenter Trial." *JAAD* 34.3 (1996) 482–85.

Shalita, Alan R. "Topical Antimicrobials in Acne Therapy." Presented at AAD annual meeting, New Orleans, La., 26 February 2002.

———. "The Role of Retinoids in Treating Acne." Presented at AAD annual meeting, Orlando, Fla., 27 February 1998.

Sullivan, Michele G. "Abandon Antibiotics in Battle Against *P. acnes*." *S&A News* 34.5 (2003): 19.

Thiboutot, Diane M. "Acne 1991–2001." *JAAD* 47.1 (2002): 109–17.

———. "Acne and Rosacea: New and Emerging Therapies." *Derm Clinics* 18.1 (2000): 63–71.

———. "Acne Therapies for the Future?" Presented at AAD annual meeting, New Orleans, La., 26 February 2002.

Walsh, Nancy. "Active Acne Cleared with Four Laser Treatments." *S&A News* 33.6 (2002): 1–3.

Webster, Guy F. "Topical Tretinoin in Acne Therapy." *JAAD* 39.2 (1998): S38–44.

Chapter 7: Accutane

Berson, Diane. "Acne Therapy: Safety Issues." Presented at AAD annual meeting, Orlando, Fla., 27 February 1998.

Bull, Jonca. Statement before the Committee on Government Reform, U.S. House of Representatives, 5 December 2000.

"Controversies in the Use of Isotretinoin: A Clinical Perspective." *S&A News* (Supplement, 2000).

Hobson, Katherine. "Mind versus Face." *U.S. News and World Report* (1 April 2002).

Jancin, Bruce. "Intermittent Isotretinoin Good for Older Patients." *S&A News* 33.1 (2002): 31.

Jick, Susan, H. M. Kremers, and C. Vasilakis-Scaramozza. "Isotretinoin Use and Risk of Depression, Psychotic Symptoms, Suicide and Attempted Suicide." *Arch Derm* 136 (2000): 1231–36.

Lamberg, Lynne. "Acne Drug Depression Warnings Highlight Need for Expert Care." *JAMA* 279 (1998): 1057.

Leyden, James. "The Role of Isotretinoin in the Treatment of Acne: Personal Observations." *JAAD* 39.2 (1998): S45–49.

Lookingbill, Donald P. "Isotretinoin: Formulation and Dosing Strategies." Presented at AAD annual meeting, New Orleans, La., 26 February 2002.

Lowenstein, Eve J. "Isotretinoin Made SMART and Simple." *Cutis* 70 (2002): 115–20.

Meadows, Michelle. "The Power of Accutane: The Benefits and Risks of a Breakthrough Acne Drug." *FDA Consumer Magazine* (March–April 2002).

Mechcatie, Elizabeth. "Low IQ Seen in Kids Exposed to Accutane in Utero." *S&A News* 29.7 (1997).

——. "Studies Highlight Limitations of Accutane PPP." *S&A News* 32.10 (2001): 6.

———. "Feds Debate Tighter Grip on Accutane." *S&A News* 34.1 (2003): 1.

Oberemok, Steve S., and Alan R. Shalita. "The Pros and Cons of Oral Therapy for Acne." *S&A* 9.9 (2001).

Peck, Gary L., T. G. Olsen, F. W. Yoder, et al. "Prolonged Remissions of Cystic and Conglabate Acne with 13-cis-retinoic Acid." *NEJM* 300 (1979): 329–33.

"Psychiatric Adverse Events in Isotretinoin-Treated Patients." *S&A News* (Supplement, 2001).

Scarbeck, Kathy. "Intermittent Isotretinoin Benefits Some Adult Acne." *S&A News* 29.5 (1997).

Strauss, John S. "Isotretinoin: Update on Issues." Presented at AAD annual meeting, New Orleans, La., 26 February 2002.

Thiboutot, Diane M. "Safety Issues in Isotretinoin Therapy." Presented at AAD annual meeting, Washington, D.C., 4 March 2001.

Webster, Guy F. "Isotretinoin Resistance?" Presented at AAD annual meeting, New Orleans, La., 26 February 2002.

Wysowski, D. K., M. Pitts, and J. Beitz. "An Analysis of Reports of Depression and Suicide in Patients Treated with Isotretinoin." *JAMA* 45 (2001): 515–19.

Chapter 8: Hormones and Hormonal Treatment

Berson, Diane. "Hormones and Acne: Clinical Evaluation and Management." Presented at AAD annual meeting, Washington, D.C., 6 March 2001.

Danby, William F. "Hormonal Influences in Acne." Presented at AAD annual meeting, Washington, D.C., 4 March 2001.

DeMott, Kathryn. "OC Use Cuts Facial Acne Lesion Count by Half." *S&A News* 32.7 (2001): 18.

Gutman, Cheryl. "Studies Confirm Low-Dose Contraceptive Treats Acne Effectively." *Derm Times* (1 June 2001).

Leyden, James, et al. "Efficacy of a Low-Dose Oral Contraceptive Containing 20 ug of Ethinyl Estradiol and 100 ug of Levonorgestrel for the Treatment of Moderate Acne: A Randomized, Placebo-Controlled Trial." *JAAD* 47.3 (2002): 399–409.

Lucky, Anne W. "Acne & Polycystic Ovary Syndrome." Presented at AAD annual meeting, New Orleans, La., 26 February 2002.

———. "Acne: A Marker for Other Medical Problems?" Presented at AAD annual meeting, San Francisco, Calif., 11 March 2000.

———. "Hormonal Treatment of Acne." Presented at AAD annual meeting, Orlando, Fla., 27 February 1998.

Maleskey, G., M. Kittel, and the Editors of Prevention Health Books for Women. *The Hormone Connection.* Emmaus, Pa.: Rodale, 2001.

Plewig, Gerd. "Adrenogenital Syndrome in Difficult to Manage Acne Patients." Presented at AAD annual meeting, Washington, D.C., 4 March 2001.

Schwartz, Erika. *The Hormone Solution.* New York: Warner Books, 2002.

Shaw, James C. "Low-Dose Adjunctive Spironolactone in the Treatment of Acne in Women." *JAAD* 43.3 (2000): 498–502.

———. "Acne Briefs." Vol. 3, no. 2, 2002. Available at http://www.academymedpublish.com/Acne_Briefs/ACNEv3n2.txt.

Thiboutot, Diane. "Oral Contraceptives: Update for Dermatologists." Presented at AAD annual meeting, San Francisco, Calif., 11 March 2000.

———. "The Role of Hormones in Acne." Presented at AAD annual meeting, Orlando, Fla., 27 February 1998.

Trickey, Ruth. *Women, Hormones and the Menstrual Cycle.* St. Leonards, NSW: Unwin Hyman, 1998.

Chapter 9: Herbs, Homeopathy, and Other Alternatives

Basset, I. B., D. L. Pannowitz, and R. S. Barnetson. "A Comparative Study of Tea-Tree Oil versus Benzoyl Peroxide in the Treatment of Acne." *Med J Australia* 153 (1990): 455.

Baumann, L. "Cosmeceutical Critique: Tea Tree Oil." *S&A News* 8.1 (2002): 14.

———. "Cosmeceutical Critique: Soy and Its Isoflavones." *S&A News* 32.8 (2001): 17.

Bedi, Monica K., and P. D. Shenfelt. "Herbal Therapy in Dermatology." *Arch Derm* 138 (2002): 232–42.

Chu, Anthony, and Anne Lovell. *The Good Skin Doctor: A Leading Dermatologist's Guide to Beating Acne.* London: Thorsons, 1999.

Cordain, L., et al. "Acne Vulgaris: A Disease of Western Civilization." *Arch Derm* 138 (2002): 1584–90.

Draelos, Zoe Diana. "Adding Vitamins to the Mix: Skin Care Products That Can Benefit the Skin." Press conference at AAD annual meeting, San Francisco, Calif., 11 March 2000.

Hoffmann, David. "Acne." Available from http://www.healthy.net.

Internet Health Library. "Acupuncture and Acne." Available from http://www.internethealthlibrary.com/Health-problems/Acne.

Jaknin, Jeanette. *Smart Medicine for Your Skin.* New York: Avery, 2001.

Levin, Cheryl, and H. Maibach. "Exploration of 'Alternative' and 'Natural' Drugs in Dermatology." *Arch Derm* 138 (2002): 207–11.

Murray, Michael, and Joseph Pizzorno. *Encyclopedia of Natural Medicine.* New York: Prima Publishing, 1998.

PDR for Non-Prescription Drugs and Dietary Supplements. Montvale, N.J.: Medical Economics Company, 2001.

Perricone, Nicholas. *The Acne Prescription.* New York: HarperCollins, 2003.

Roberts, Arthur J., Mary E. O'Brien, and Genell Subak-Sharpe. *Nutraceuticals.* New York: Berkley Publishing Group, 2001.

Shalita, A. R., J. G. Smith, L. C. Parish, et al. "Topical Nicotinamide Compared with Clindamycin in the Treatment of Inflammatory Acne Vulgaris." *Int J Derm* 34.6 (1995): 434–37.

Tanweer, A. Syed, and A. Qureshi Zulfiqar. "Treatment of Acne Vulgaris with 2% Polyphenone (Epigallocatechin Gallate or Green Tea Extract) in Cream." Poster at AAD annual meeting, Washington, D.C., March 2001.

Time-Life Books. *The Medical Advisor.* 2d edition. Alexandria: Time-Life Books, 2002.

Trattner, Elizabeth. "Alternative Medicine." In *Cosmetic Dermatology: Principles and Practice.* New York: McGraw-Hill, 2002: 125–35.

Chapter 10: The Mind-Skin Connection

Baldwin, Hillary E. "The Relationship Between Acne Vulgaris and the Psyche." *Cutis* 70.2 (2002): 133–39.

Chiu, Annie, S. Y. Chon, and A. B. Kimball. "The Response of Skin Disease to Stress: Changes in the Severity of Acne Vulgaris as Affected by Examination Stress." *Arch Derm* 139.7 (2003).

Goldman, Erik L. "Where the Psyche Meets the Soma." *S&A News* 33.4 (2002): 1.

Grossbart, Ted A., and Carl S. Sherman. *Skin Deep: A Mind-Body Program for Healthy Skin.* Santa Fe: Health Press, 1992.

Gupta, Madhulika A., and A. K. Gupta. "The Use of Psychotropic Drugs in Dermatology." *Derm Clinics* 18.4 (2000): 711–24.

Tausk, Francisco, and H. Nousari. "Stress and the Skin." *Arch Derm* 137 (2001): 78–82.

Chapter 11: Looking Good

Abramovits, William, and Aldo Gonzalez-Serva. "Sebum, Cosmetics and Skin Care." *Derm Clinics* 18.4 (2000): 617–20.

Baumann, Leslie S. "Skin Care Suggestions for Patients." *S&A News* 33.1 (2003): 35.

Cunliffe, William J. "Pathological & Pharmacological Control of Comedones." Presented at AAD annual meeting, Orlando, Fla., 27 February 1998.

Draelos, Zoe Diana. "Cosmetics and Skin Care Products," "Therapeutic Moisturizers," and "Colored Facial Cosmetics." *Derm Clinics* 18.4 (2000): 557–59, 597–607; 621–30.

———. "Cosmetic Conundrums: Why Do Sunscreens Cause Breakouts . . . ?" *Derm Times* (1 April 2003).

———. "Degradation and Migration of Facial Foundations." *JAAD* 45.4 (2001): 542–43.

Guttman, Cheryl. "Less common modalities play role in Tx." *Derm Times* (1 September 2002), supplement.

Chapter 12: Acne and Your Children

Brecher, A.R., and S. J. Orlow. "Oral Retinoid Therapy for Dermatologic Conditions in Children and Adolescents." *JAAD* 49.2 (2002): 171–82.

Finn, Robert. "Neonatal, Infantile Acne Must Be Treated Differently." *Pediatric News* 35.12 (2001): 36.

Fried, Richard. "Facts and Fiction About Teenagers and Acne." *S&A* 9.4 (2001).

Lucky, Anne W. "A Review of Infantile and Pediatric Acne." *Dermatology* 196 (1998): 95–97.

Lucky, Anne W., F. M. Biro, L. A. Simbarti, et al. "Predictors of Severity of Acne Vulgaris in Young Adolescent Girls." *J Pediatrics* 130.1 (1997): 30–39.

Tucker, Miriam E. "Neonatal Acne Actually May Not Be Acne at All." *Pediatric News* 36.8 (2002): 30.

Chapter 13: Scars and Scar Revision

Alster, Tina S. *Manual of Cutaneous Laser Techniques.* Philadelphia: Lippincott Williams and Wilkins, 2000.

Alster, Tina S., and T. McMeekin. "Improvement of Facial Acne Scars by the 585 nm Flashlamp-Pumped Pulsed Dye Laser." *JAMA* 35 (1996): 79–81.

Alster, Tina S., and Lydia Preston. *The Essential Guide to Cosmetic Laser Surgery.* New York: Alliance Publishers, 1997.

Klein, Arnold W. *Tissue Augmentation in Clinical Practice.* New York, Basel, Hong Kong: Marcel Dekker, 1998.

Orentreich, D. S., and N. Orentreich. "Subcutaneous Incisionless (Subcision) Surgery for the Correction of Depressed Scars and Wrinkles." *Derm Surgery* 21.6 (1995): 543–49.

Rosio, Timothy J. "Revision of Acne, Traumatic and Surgical Scars." In *Cutaneous Surgery.* Edited by R. Wheeland. Philadelphia: W. B. Saunders Company, 1994.

Walia, S., and T. Alster. "Prolonged Clinical and Histologic Effects from CO_2 Laser Resurfacing of Atrophic Acne Scars." *Derm Surg* 25 (1999): 926–30.

INDEX

Accutane (isotretinoin), 6, 8, 66, 69,
    74, 84, 90–105, 205
    author's experience with, 91,
        99–100
    CAM and, 126–27
    children and, 167–69, 171–74
    failures of, 104–5
    history of, 91–93
    indications for, 99–101
    side effects of, 90–91, 93–99,
        102–3, 127, 167, 171–74
    taking it, 101–4
    what it does, 93–94
Ache hunter-gatherers, 124
acne:
    attitudes toward, 13–15, 17
    author's experience with, 1–2, 6,
        91, 99–100, 163, 170–71
    causes of, 3–5, 7, 11–12, 14,
        34–45, 106–9, 111–12, 167
    complexities of, xi–xii, 7, 126
    definition of, 32–33
    formation of, 18–28, 31–33
    genetic predisposition toward,
        35–38, 145, 163–64
    in history, 4, 11
    misconceptions about, 2, 11–14
    mysteries about, 31–32
    noninflammatory, 24, 33
    persistence of, 8–9, 14
    prevalence of, xi, 2–4, 32
    seriousness of, 8, 15–17
    statistics on, xi, 2–4, 6–8, 12, 14,

        46, 87, 100, 104, 106–7, 110,
        113, 128, 133–35, 149, 165,
        177, 181, 185, 196
    talking about, 15
    in unusual locations, 65
Acne and Rosacea (Plewig and Klig-
    man), 18, 152
acne burnout, 31–32
acne conglobata, 92
acne cosmetica, 35–39
acne excoriee, 45
acneiform eruptions, 33, 161
    cosmetics and, 36, 38
acne mechanica, 45
Acne Prescription, The (Perricone),
    125
acne rosacea, 33, 65, 84–85
Acne RX (Fulton), 148, 151
acne vulgaris, 32–33, 35–36
Acnomel, 60–61, 170, 213–14
adapalene (Differin), 71–72, 75, 82,
    149
adolescents, 165–71, 173
    Accutane and, 90–91, 96, 100
    acne formation and, 20
    acne in adults vs., 2–4, 8–10
    hormones and, 106
    mind-skin connection and, 145
    and misconceptions about acne,
        11–13
    and mysteries about acne, 32
    neonatal acne and, 165–66
    OTC remedies and, 49, 55, 62

adrenal glands, 20, 41
  children and, 165–68
  disorders of, 114, 167
  hormonal acne and, 107, 109,
    112, 114
  hormonal treatments and,
    115–16, 118–19
  mind-skin connection and,
    140–41
Advil, 149–50
African Americans, 30, 75, 184
  causes of acne in, 37–38, 42
age, aging, xiii, 1–4, 41, 186
  acne formation and, 21
  CAM and, 125, 132, 134
  hormones and, 106, 110, 112,
    115
  medications and, 8, 55, 62,
    64–65, 68, 70–71, 78–79
  mind-skin connection and, 145
  and misconceptions about acne,
    11
  and mysteries about acne, 31–32
  scars and, 177, 181, 192
  see also adolescents; children
age spots, 43
Akne-Mycin, 81
alcohol, 138
  looking good and, 151, 154–55
  OTC remedies and, 52, 56, 58,
    62
  prescription treatments and, 81,
    85
aldosterone, 118–19
Alesse, 116–17
Allergan, 71
AlloDerm, 192
alpha hydroxy acids (AHAs), 58,
  68, 213
Alster, Tina, xi–xiv, 13, 175,
  183–84, 187, 193–95

alternative medicine, *see* complementary and alternative medicine
American Academy of Dermatology (AAD), 105, 156, 172
American Society for Dermatologic Surgery, 193–94
Amnesteem, 91, 96
androgens, 3, 41, 66
  acne formation and, 20
  CAM and, 124–25, 130–31
  children and, 165, 167
  hormonal acne and, 107–14
  hormonal treatments and, 115–20
  mind-skin connection and, 141
  overactive receptors for, 110
animal-derived collagen injections, 189–90
anti-androgens, 118–20
antibiotics, 8, 36, 75–84, 86–87, 100–101
  Accutane and, 100
  bacterial resistance to, 76–77, 80–81
  benzoyl peroxide in combination with, 83–84
  CAM and, 123, 126, 136
  children and, 167, 171
  comparisons between benzoyl peroxide and, 52
  looking good and, 148–49
  oral, 66, 75–81, 101, 167
  topical, 66, 73, 76, 80–81, 86, 117, 149
antioxidants, 125–26, 210
  CAM and, 126, 128–29, 131–34
  OTC remedies and, 57
Artefill, 189–90
Asians, 30, 184
aspirin, 56, 103
Autologen, 190
autologous dermal grafts, 192

autologous fat fillers, 191–92
Avage, 71
Aveeno, 132, 135, 208, 211
Avita, 69–70, 82
azelaic acid, 84, 183
Azelex, 84

bacteria, 32–33, 206–8
    acne formation and, 24–27
    CAM and, 133, 135
    and causes of acne, 42–43
    looking good and, 148–49
    and mysteries about acne, 32
    OTC remedies and, 48, 51–54,
        59–61
    prescription treatments and, 66,
        68, 76–78, 80–87, 93, 101
Basis, 206
Baumann, Leslie, 155
Begoun, Paula, 155, 205
benzoyl peroxide, 47–48, 50–56,
        60, 206–10
    in acne regimens, 63–64
    advantages of, 51–53
    CAM and, 133–35, 138
    children and, 166–67, 170–71
    looking good and, 148–49
    prescription treatments and, 52,
        70–71, 73, 75, 77, 82–84, 136
    side effects of, 53–55, 58
    use of, 53–55
Bergfeld, Wilma:
    CAM and, 126–27, 130
    hormones and, 107, 112
Bershad, Susan, 12–13
    CAM and, 122
    looking good and, 154
    on OTC remedies, 61–64
    prescription treatments and, 66,
        71, 73–74, 77
Berson, Diane, 100–101, 104–5

beta hydroxy acid (BHA), 56
Bioré, 132, 208
birth control pills, 16, 109
    in hormonal treatments, 116–19
    prescription treatments and, 66,
        78, 89
birthmarks, 14
blackheads, 3, 39
    acne formation and, 18, 22–24,
        26
    CAM and, 134
    children and, 165–66, 168–69
    extraction of, 152–54
    and misconceptions about acne, 12
    OTC remedies and, 55, 65
    prescription treatments and, 55,
        67
bleeding, blood, bloodstream, blood
        vessels, 20
    acne formation and, 27
    CAM and, 124–25, 129
    hormones and, 108, 113, 115–16
    looking good and, 148, 150–52
    prescription treatments and, 78,
        94, 99
    scars and, 28, 184–85
blue light treatment (ClearLight), 87
botanicals, 210
    anti-inflammatory, 132–33
    OTC remedies and, 49–50
breakouts, 73
    Accutane and, 100–101
    acne formation and, 21
    of author, 1–2
    hormones and, 109–11, 115,
        117–18
    mind-skin connection and, 144
    and misconceptions about acne,
        11–12
    premenstrual, see premenstrual
        acne

Brody, Harold, 153, 177–81, 185–86, 193–94
Brown, Bobbi, 10, 159–62
Burgess, Cheryl, 38
Burt's Bees, 136

cadaver tissue implants, 192
calcium deposits, 62–63
camouflage, 159–60, 162
Camp Discovery, 13
Centers for Disease Control, 94
Cetaphil, 81, 206
    retinoids and, 72, 75–76
cheeks, 37, 45, 72
    children and, 165
    scars and, 175, 192
chemical acne (occupational acne), 39–40
chemical peels, 104, 177, 180–83
chemotactic factors, 25
children, 163–74
    Accutane and, 167–69, 171–74
    skin and, 11, 163–66, 168, 170–71
    see also adolescents
chin, 28, 31, 45, 72, 165, 175
chocolate, 12, 16, 123
choracne, 40
Chu, Anthony, 138
Clean & Clear, 132, 205, 207–8, 210–12
cleansers, cleansing, 205–7
    acne formation and, 20–22, 25
    children and, 169–71
    OTC remedies and, 62–64, 206–7
    prescription treatments and, 72, 75–76, 83, 103
Clearasil, 205, 208–12, 213
ClearLight (blue light treatment), 87
Clenia, 85
Cleocin T, 81

climate, 44
Clinac, 83, 155, 214
Clindagel, 81
clindamycin, 81, 86
Clinique, 49–50, 52, 132, 205, 208–9, 212
clothing, 44–45
coal-tar acne, 40
cocoa butter, 38
collagen:
    and acne in skin of color, 30
    CAM and, 129
    prescription treatments and, 70, 72
    scars and, 29, 176–84, 186, 189–91
collagen remodeling, 179–84, 186
colonial women, 4–5
color, 159–60
comedones, 207, 210, 213
    acne formation and, 21–27, 32–33
    and causes of acne, 35–40, 43–45
    children and, 165–66
    closed, see whiteheads
    hormones and, 110
    looking good and, 150–54
    mysteries about, 31–32
    open, see blackheads
    OTC remedies and, 46, 48, 51–52, 55–56, 58, 60
    prescription treatments and, 66–69, 71, 73, 77, 79, 82, 85, 93, 101, 153
    scars and, 29
    secondary, 27–28, 101
    surgery and, 101–2
complementary and alternative medicine (CAM), xii, 121–38
    and diet, 122–26, 129, 134

and herbal treatments, 89, 122, 130–33, 203
and homeopathy, 137–38
and nutritional supplements, 89, 125–30, 203
and pregnancy, 127, 203
and TCM, 137
and topical treatments, 131–36
congenital adrenal hyperplasia (CAH), 114, 167
Cordain, Loren, 124
corpus luteum, 113
Cortaid, 150
corticosteroids, 118, 147–48
cortisol, 140–41, 146
cortisone, 150
cosmetics, xii, 10, 33–39, 89
   acne formation and, 18, 20
   CAM and, 126, 131, 133
   and causes of acne, 34–39
   looking good and, 154–55, 157–62
   medications and, 8, 47, 49, 51, 53, 71, 81
   scars and, 187–88, 190–92
   and seriousness of acne, 17
CosmoDerm, 190
CosmoPlast, 190
Couric, Katie, 13–14
Cunliffe, William J., 89, 100, 103
Cushing's syndrome, 114
Cymetra, 192
cyproterone acetate, 119
cysts, xiii, 27–29, 37
   acne formation and, 24, 27–28
   CAM and, 123
   children and, 167
   hormones and, 112–13, 115, 117
   prescription treatments and, 86–87, 92, 99
   scars and, 28–29

Dahl, Mark V., 13
dairy foods, 123, 125–26
Dapsone (sulfones), 86
dark skin:
   CAM and, 135
   looking good and, 156, 159
   retinoids and, 73–76
   scars and, 183–84, 186
   see also skin of color
Dattner, Alan, 122–26
DDF, 205, 207–9, 213
deep peels, 104, 181–83
dehydroepiandrosterone (DHEA), 41–42
dehydroepiandrosterone sulfate (DHEA-S), 114
Depo-Provera, 117
depression, 142, 145
   Accutane and, 90, 97–99, 172–74
   inner scars and, 196
dermabrasion, 104, 177, 179–82, 184–86
dermatitis:
   contact, 136
   perioral, 33, 65
   seborrheic, 59
dermatologists, 64–65
dermis, 27–30
   acne formation and, 27–28
   prescription treatments and, 70
   scars and, 29, 176, 179–82, 184, 186, 191–92
Diane, 119
Dianette, 119
diet, 20
   CAM and, 122–26, 129, 134
   hormones and, 109
   mind-skin connection and, 142
   and misconceptions about acne, 11–12, 14

diet *(cont.)*
  prescription treatments and,
    78–80
  and seriousness of acne, 16
Differin (adapalene), 71–72, 75, 81,
    149
dihydrotestosterone (DHT), 20
  CAM and, 129, 131, 133
  hormonal acne and, 108–9
  hormonal treatments and, 115,
    119–20
Dilantin, 40, 105
Dove, 64, 206
doxycycline, 79
Draelos, Zoe Diana, 156–57,
    160–61

eczema, 14, 81, 136, 140
embarrassment, 14–18
emotions, xi–xiii, 11–13
  Accutane and, 100, 173
  and causes of acne, 5, 34–35
  inner scars and, 196, 199
  mind-skin connection and, 140,
    142–43
  and misconceptions about acne,
    12–13
  and seriousness of acne, 16–17
epidermis, 43, 64–65
  acne formation and, 22–23, 27
  looking good and, 152
  prescription treatments and, 88
  scars and, 176, 179–80, 182,
    186, 192
erythromycin, 80–81, 136, 167
Estée Lauder, 50, 132
estrogen, 108, 111–12, 134
  and causes of acne, 41
  hormonal treatments and, 118
Estrostep, 116–17
Eucerin, 206

exercise, 143–44, 197–98
exfoliants, exfoliation, 68
  looking good and, 154
  OTC remedies and, 48, 50,
    55–58, 62–63, 207, 210
  scars and, 180, 183

face, facial foundations, 154
  Accutane and, 92, 104
  looking good and, 157–62
  scars and, 182, 192
fascia injections (Fascian), 190–91
fats, fatty acids, 20, 125, 134
  acne formation and, 25
  OTC remedies and, 51–52
fibroblasts, 30, 180
fillers:
  implanted, 187–88, 192–93
  injected, 187–92
  scars and, 177–78, 187–94
Finacea, 84
finasteride, 120
Finevin, 84
5-alpha reductase:
  CAM and, 129, 131, 133
  hormonal acne and, 108, 110,
    115, 119–20
5-alpha reductase inhibitors, 120
Flagyl, 85
flares, *see* breakouts
flutamide, 119–20
folic acid, 86
follicle stimulating hormone (FSH),
    131
folliculitis, 33, 36, 42, 165
Food and Drug Administration
    (FDA), 16, 38, 41, 43, 201
  and CAM, 127, 130, 136, 138
  and hormonal treatments, 117
  and OTC remedies, 47, 49–51
  and prescription treatments,

69–71, 85–87, 91, 94, 96–99,
172–73
and scars, 188
forehead, 31, 37–38, 72, 165
free radicals, 29–30
Fried, Richard, 140, 142–46, 174,
196–99
Fulton, James, 123, 148, 151
fungi, 33, 59

Galderma, 81
Glogau, Richard, 178, 188–93
glycolic acid, 58, 213
looking good and, 154
prescription treatments and, 75
scars and, 180, 183
gonadotropins, 41, 116
granulomous response, 189
green tea extract, 133
guilt, 13, 144

Hahnemann, Samuel, 137
hair follicles, 18–29, 33
acne formation and, 18–28
hormones and, 109
scars and, 29
see also sebaceous follicles
Hebra, Ferdinand, 4
herbs, herbal treatments, 49, 89,
122, 130–33, 203, 210
hexachlorophene, 52
hippie acne, 45
Hispanics, 30, 75, 184
Hoffmann-La Roche, 92
homeopathy, 137–38
hormone replacement therapy, 109,
112
hormones, xiii, 3, 10, 66, 68, 78,
105–20
Accutane and, 105
acne formation and, 20–21

CAM and, 124–25, 128–31,
133–34, 137
and causes of acne, 34–35,
40–41, 106–9
children and, 165, 167–68
and medical conditions leading
to acne, 112–15, 117
mind-skin connection and,
140–41, 143–44, 146
in normal life, 110–12
OTC remedies and, 48
treatments with, 84, 106–7,
114–20, 203
human collagen injections, 190
hyaluronic acid fillers, 191
hydrogen peroxide, 52
hygiene, 12, 14
hyperpigmentation, 29–30
CAM and, 134–35
looking good and, 156
prescription treatments and, 75,
84
scars and, 182–83

ibuprofen, 149–50
ice cubes, 148–51
ichthyosis, 168
immune system, 41, 43
acne formation, 25–26
mind-skin connection and,
142–43
impetigo, 45
implanted fillers, 187–88, 192–93
infantile acne, 164, 166–68
inflammation, inflammations, 210
CAM and, 125, 128–29, 131–37
children and, 166–67, 169–71
looking good and, 147–50, 152,
156
mind-skin connection and,
140–41, 143

inflammation, inflammations *(cont.)*
 OTC remedies and, 48, 50,
  56–57, 59–61
 prescription treatments and,
  66–68, 71, 75–77, 79–81,
  83–87, 93, 101–2
 scars and, 176
injected fillers, 187–92
insulin resistance, 113–15
isolutrol, 133–34
isoniazid, 41
isotretinoin, *see* Accutane

Jacknin, Jeanette, 128–29
jawline, 28, 31, 115, 175
Joey, 205, 211
Johnson & Johnson, 132, 135
*Journal of the American Academy of
 Dermatology,* 160

keloids, 30
keratinocytes:
 acne formation and, 22, 24
 CAM and, 127
 OTC remedies and, 55
 prescription treatments and, 68
Ketsugo, 133
Kiavan Islanders, 124
Klear Action, 209
Kligman, Albert M., 3–5, 7–9,
  17–18
 acne formation and, 18, 31–32
 CAM and, 123
 looking good and, 152
 on OTC remedies, 55, 59
 prescription treatments and, 67,
  100
knowledge, 9–11, 17
 inner scars and, 197
 mind-skin connection and, 145
Korean War, 44

lactation, 34, 165
 hormones and, 106, 111
 prescription treatments and, 74,
  78–80
lasers, xii
 CO_2, 183–84, 186–87
 Erbium, 183–84, 186
 nonablative, 88, 186–87
 resurfacing, 88, 104, 175, 177,
  181–84, 186–87, 194
 Smoothbeam, 88, 186
Leno, Jay, 15–16
Leyden, James, 67–68, 91
light therapy, 86–88
lips, lip balms, 37, 103
Liquimat, 213–14
lithium, 40, 78
looking good, 147–62
 camouflage and, 159–60, 162
 color and, 159–60
 and extracting blackheads and
  whiteheads, 152–54
 facial foundations and, 157–62
 makeup migration and, 160–62
 moisturizers and, 156
 oil blotters and, 154–55, 162
 popping pimples and, 150–51
 spot treatments and, 147–51,
  160
 sunscreens and, 155–57, 161
luteinizing hormone (LH), 111, 131

macrolines, 77, 80
macules, 28–29
 looking good and, 156
 pigmented, 29
 scars and, 28
magnesium hydroxide, 154–55
makeup, *see* cosmetics
makeup migration, 160–62
Malassezia sympodialis, 165

Mallorca acne, 44
medications, 4–11
    abundance of, 5–8, 10
    CAM and, 122, 126–27
    children and, 164–74
    hormonal treatments and, 84,
        106–7, 114–20, 203
    looking good and, 147–50,
        153–54
    patients' knowledge about, 9–11
    side effects of, xiii, 8, 53–55, 58,
        67–69, 74, 78–81, 83, 86, 88–
        99, 102–3, 118–19, 122, 127,
        134–35, 167, 171–74, 201–2
    see also over-the-counter reme-
        dies; prescription treatments
melanin:
    acne formation and, 23
    and acne in skin of color, 29–30
    CAM and, 134
    looking good and, 159
    prescription treatments and, 84
melanocytes, 29–30
    scars and, 182, 184
menopause, xiii, 2, 34, 106, 111–12
menstruation, 5
    Accutane and, 102
    hormones and, xiii, 34, 106,
        109–10, 113, 115, 117
    and misconceptions about acne,
        12
    and seriousness of acne, 16–17
metronidazole, 85
microcomedones:
    acne formation and, 23, 26, 32
    mind-skin connection and, 141
    OTC remedies and, 48, 61
    prescription treatments and, 68,
        73
microdermabrasion, 180
milia, 33, 165

milk of magnesia, 155
mind-skin connection, 139–46
    hormones and, 140–41, 143–44,
        146
    taking control and, 143–45
    vicious cycle in, 141–43
minocycline, 79–80, 149
moisturizers:
    CAM and, 135
    looking good and, 156
    OTC remedies and, 62
    prescription treatments and, 73,
        76, 85, 89, 103
Murad Acne, 205, 208, 211, 213

National Institutes of Health
    (NIH), 92–94
Nature's Cure, 138, 209
neck, 31, 182
neonatal acne, 164–66
neonatal cephalic pustulosis, 165
Neutrogena, 4, 52, 54, 132, 205–9,
    211–12
neutrophils, 136, 149
    acne formation, 25–27
    OTC remedies and, 52
New England Journal of Medicine, 92
niacin, 86, 126, 128
niacinamide, 134
nicotinamide (Nicomide), 86
Nieman, Erin, 57
nodules, 26–29, 37
    acne formation and, 24, 26–28
    children and, 167
    hormones and, 110
    prescription treatments and, 75,
        92, 99–100
    scars and, 28–29
Noritate, 85
Norplant, 117
Novacet, 85

nutritional supplements, 89, 109,
    125–30, 203

obesity, 14
O'Brien, Conan, 16
occupational acne (chemical acne),
    39–40
O'Donoghue, Marianne, 2
    and causes of acne, 37, 39, 44–45
    looking good and, 148
    mind-skin connection and, 139,
        141
    on OTC remedies, 51, 55, 60,
        62–64
    prescription treatments and, 82
oil, 214
    acne formation and, 19–21,
        23–26
    and causes of acne, 39–40, 43, 45
    children and, 165
    hormones and, 109, 115, 118
    looking good and, 147, 154–55,
        157–62
    OTC remedies and, 48–50,
        54–55, 58, 62
    prescription treatments and, 66,
        73, 75, 77, 81, 83, 101, 103
    production of, 20–21
oil acne, 40
oil blotters, 154–55, 162
Olay, 132, 134, 206
Oreal, L', 208, 211–12
Ortho Tri-Cyclen, 116–17
ovaries, 20, 95, 111–17, 137
    children and, 168
    hormones and, 107–9, 111–13,
        115–17, 119, 131
    tumors of, 114–15
over-the-counter (OTC) remedies,
    xiii, 4–6, 46–65, 89, 205–14
    abundance of, 5–6, 10

Accutane and, 103
acne-fighting ingredients in,
    47–49
AHAs and, 58, 68, 213
children and, 166–67, 169–71
dermatologists and, 64–65
extra, added ingredients in,
    49–51
looking good and, 149–50,
    153–54
mind-skin connection and, 144
pregnancy and, 203
for prevention, 61
primer on use of, 61–63
regimens for, 63–64
side effects of, 53–55, 58,
    134–35
see also benzoyl peroxide; com-
    plementary and alternative
    medicine; salicylic acid
ovulation:
    and causes of acne, 34
    hormones and, 34, 106, 110,
        112–13, 116
Oxy, 62, 170–71, 205, 207, 209–10

pantothenic acid, 128
papules, 30, 33
    acne formation and, 24, 26–28
    CAM and, 134
    children and, 166, 170
    hormones and, 111
    looking good and, 149, 157, 161
    OTC remedies and, 51
    prescription treatments and, 67,
        75, 85
Papulex, 134
Paula's Choice, 155, 205–6, 209,
    211–12
Peck, Gary L., 92
penicillin, 77, 91

perimenopause, 111–12
Periostat, 79
Perricone, Nicholas, 124–25,
    131–32
Peter Thomas Roth, 205, 207–10,
    213–14
phantom acne, 196–97
Philosophy, 212
pHisohex, pHisoderm, 52, 205,
    208, 212
photo-rejuvination, 186
photosensitizing agents, 73–74
picking, 45, 61
pilosebaceous units:
    acne formation and, 18–19
    hormones and, 109
    scars and, 182
pimples, 3
    Accutane and, 100
    acne formation and, 18, 23–28
    CAM and, 124, 135
    and causes of acne, 36–37, 39,
        42, 45
    children and, 163–64, 168
    hormones and, 109
    looking good and, 147–51, 158
    mind-skin connection and, 139,
        141, 146
    OTC remedies and, 46, 51–52,
        56, 61–62
    popping, 150–51
    scars and, 29
pituitary, 41, 109, 111, 115–16, 131
Plewig, Gerd, 36, 45
    Accutane and, 103
    acne formation and, 18, 28, 31
    CAM and, 123
    children and, 164, 168–69, 171
    looking good and, 152
    mind-skin connection and, 139
    on OTC remedies, 51, 60

Plexion, 85
Polis, Laurie, 2, 7–8, 40, 42–43, 72,
    156, 173
polycystic ovary syndrome (PCOS),
    112–13, 117, 137
pores:
    acne formation and, 19, 21–24
    blockage of, 21–23
    and causes of acne, 44–45
    looking good and, 151–52, 158
    OTC remedies and, 48–49, 62–63
    prescription treatments and,
        71–72
pore strips, 152, 154
precursor lesions, 23, 48, 68
pregnancy, 120
    CAM and, 127, 203
    hormones and, xiii, 34, 106, 111,
        113, 118, 125, 203
    prescription treatments and, 74,
        78–80, 90, 94–97, 102–3,
        201–2
premenstrual acne, 110–11, 117
    CAM and, 128, 131
    mind-skin connection and, 144
prescription treatments, xiii, 6, 10,
    59–61, 64–89, 101–3, 188
    acne caused or aggravated by,
        40–41
    array of, 66
    benzoyl peroxide and, 52,
        70–71, 73, 75, 77, 82–84, 136
    CAM and, 136
    children and, 166–74
    comparisons between OTC
        remedies and, 46, 52, 55,
        60–61, 65
    hormonal treatments and, 84,
        106–7, 114–20, 203
    light therapy in, 86–88
    looking good and, 149–50, 153–54

prescription treatments (cont.)
mind-skin connection and, 144–45
pitfalls in use of, 88–89
side effects of, 67–69, 74, 78–81,
83, 86, 88–99, 102–3, 127,
167, 171–74, 201–2
see also Accutane; antibiotics;
retinoids
pressure, 44–45
Pride, Howard, 164, 166–68,
170–71, 174
Proactiv, 5, 53, 170–71, 205, 207,
209, 213–14
Procter & Gamble, 132, 134
progesterone, 108, 113, 116, 125
progestin, 116–17, 119
Propionibacterium acnes (P. acnes),
206–8
acne formation and, 25–26
CAM and, 135
and causes of acne, 43
looking good and, 148
and mysteries about acne, 32
OTC remedies and, 48, 51–54, 61
prescription treatments and,
76–77, 80, 82, 84, 86–87, 93,
101
psoriasis, 14, 42, 65, 71, 140
psychotherapy, 15, 145, 196, 198
Purpose, 206
pustules, 32–33, 38
acne formation and, 23–24, 27
CAM and, 134
children and, 165–66, 169–70
looking good and, 150, 154, 157,
161
and mysteries about acne, 32
OTC remedies and, 52
prescription treatments and, 67,
85
pyridoxine, 128

rectal cancer, 13–14
Reese, Vail, 9
Renova, 69–71
resorcinol:
looking good and, 149
in OTC remedies, 47–48, 59–60
retention hyperkeratosis, 22–23
Retin-A, 8–9, 55, 59–60, 67, 69–70,
82, 87, 127, 148
children and, 166
patients' knowledge about, 9
use of, 72
Retin-A Micro, 70, 82, 155
retinoic acid (tretinoin), 59, 63,
69–71, 81–82, 155
retinoids, 81–82, 84, 87
children and, 166–71
dark skin and, 73–76
looking good and, 153–54
options for, 69–72
oral, 74, 90–105
side effects of, 67–69, 74
synthetic, 69, 71, 82
topical, 66–77, 92, 100–101, 117,
127, 153–54, 166–71, 205
use of, 72–74
retinol (vitamin A), 67, 74, 92–94,
103, 126–27, 129
in OTC remedies, 59–60
Rezamid, 213–14
Roaccutane, 91
Roche Pharmaceuticals, 91, 96–97
Rodan, Katie, 5
Rosac, 85
rosacea, 33, 65, 84–85
Rosula, 85

salicylic acid, 47–50, 55–58, 68,
206–7, 210–13
in acne regimens, 63–64
children and, 166, 169–70

looking good and, 149, 153–54
retinoids and, 73, 75
selecting products with, 56–57
Sarnoff, Deborah, 9
saw palmetto, 131
scars, scarring, xi–xiii, 5, 8, 13,
    15–16, 28–30, 65, 174–99
    Accutane and, 91, 99–101, 104,
        174
    acne formation and, 24
    and acne in skin of color, 30
    atrophic, 176–77
    CAM and, 123
    and causes of acne, 40
    children and, 164, 166–69, 171,
        174
    full-thickness, 176
    hypertrophic, 30, 176
    inner, 196–99
    looking good and, 150–51, 158,
        162
    and mysteries about acne, 32
    revision of, xii–xiii, 175, 177–95
    and seriousness of acne, 16
    and talking about acne, 15
Schaumberg Extractor, 153–54
sebaceous follicles, 206–7, 213
    acne formation and, 19–28
    CAM and, 125, 127–28
    and causes of acne, 34–35, 40,
        42–45, 106
    children and, 165
    hormones and, 106–7, 110
    looking good and, 152–53, 161
    mind-skin connection and, 141,
        145–46
    mysteries about, 31–32
    OTC remedies and, 48, 51–52,
        56, 58, 62
    prescription treatments and,
        68–69, 72, 77, 80, 86, 88, 93

sebaceous glands, 11
    acne formation and, 19–20, 24
    CAM and, 123–24, 133
    and causes of acne, 37
    hormones and, 105, 108–9, 111,
        115
    mind-skin connection and, 141
    prescription treatments and, 83,
        88, 93, 103, 105
Seban, 155, 214
seborrhea, 20
sebum:
    acne formation and, 19–23,
        25–27
    CAM and, 127–29, 133
    and causes of acne, 36, 42
    children and, 166, 168
    hormonal treatments and,
        115–20
    looking good and, 154–55,
        161–62
    and mysteries about acne, 32
    OTC remedies and, 48, 54–55,
        61
    prescription treatments and, 83,
        88, 93, 101, 104
selenium, 129
Self, 46
sex, sexuality, 142
    Accutane and, 95–96
    and misconceptions about acne,
        11–12
sex hormone binding globulin
    (SHBG), 108, 113–16
Shalita, Alan:
    CAM and, 123
    and causes of acne, 35
    children and, 169
    looking good and, 149–50
    on OTC remedies, 46, 52,
        57–58, 61–62, 64

Shalita, Alan (cont.)
    prescription treatments and, 67–70, 77, 87, 89, 98
shame:
    and attitudes toward acne, 13–14
    mind-skin connection and, 144–45
Silverman, Robert, 153, 169–71, 174
skin, 6
    acne formation and, 18–28
    CAM and, 121, 126–29, 132–37
    and causes of acne, 34, 36–42, 44–45
    children and, 11, 163–66, 168, 170–71
    hormones and, 10, 105–12, 114–16, 118
    inner scars and, 196–97
    looking good and, 147–48, 150–52, 154–62
    and misconceptions about acne, 11–12
    OTC remedies and, 48, 52, 54–56, 58–60, 62–63, 65
    prescription treatments and, 67–76, 78, 80–84, 86–89, 92–93, 99–101, 103–4, 174
    proactive care for, 144
    scars and, 175–77, 179–87, 190–93
    and seriousness of acne, 17
    see also mind-skin connection
Skin and Allergy News, 155
skin cancers, 43, 64–65, 87
skin of color:
    acne in, 29–30
    and OTC remedies, 60
Sloan Survey, 96–97
Smart Medicine for Your Skin (Jacknin), 128
Smoothbeam laser, 88, 186

soaps, see cleansers, cleansing
sodium sulfacetimide, 61, 85
Sonya Dakar, 61
soy, 134–35
specialists, 193–95
spironolactone, 118–19
spot treatments, 208–9, 213
    children and, 170
    looking good and, 147–51, 160
squeezing, 45
steroids, 108
    acne stimulated by, 41–42
    in prescription treatments, 101
stratum corneum, 43
stress:
    and causes of acne, 4–5, 35
    hormones and, 109
    inner scars and, 197
    mind-skin connection and, 139–41, 143–46
    and misconceptions about acne, 12
Stridex, 209, 212
Stupak, Bart, 173
subcutis, 176–77
Sulfacet, 85
sulfones (Dapsone), 86
sulfur:
    children and, 170
    looking good and, 149
    in OTC remedies, 47–48, 59–61, 213
    prescription treatments and, 85
Summers Laboratory, 103
sunlight, sun damage, sun exposure, 29, 180–81
    acne caused by, 43
    CAM and, 133–34
    children and, 166
    prescription treatments and, 68, 70–71, 73–74, 78, 80

scars and, 181, 183
see also ultraviolet light
sunscreens:
looking good and, 155–57, 161
prescription treatments and, 73,
76, 85, 89, 103
surgery, xii–xiii, 65
Accutane and, 101–2, 104
looking good and, 153
see also lasers
surgical excision, 178–79
sweat, sweat glands, 21, 33, 44
synthetic implants, 193
System to Manage Accutane-
Related Teratogenicity
(SMART), 96–97
System to Prevent Isotretinoin-
Related Issues of Teratogenicity (SPIRIT), 96

Taylor, Susan, 30, 42, 75
tazarotene (Tazorac), 55, 71–72,
75–76, 82, 143
tea tree oil, 135–36
temples, 37–38
terminal follicles, 19
testes, 20, 165, 167–68
testosterone:
acne formation and, 20
CAM and, 128–29, 131, 133
and causes of acne, 41
hormonal acne and, 106, 108,
110–14
hormonal treatments and, 116–20
tetracyclines, 77–81, 126, 167
second-generation, 77, 79–80
topical, 81
titanium dioxide, 157
Today, 13–14
Traditional Chinese Medicine
(TCM), 137

treatments:
alternative, xii, 89, 121–38, 203
failure of, 7–9
hormonal, 84, 106–7, 114–20,
203
looking good and, 147–50
and misconceptions about acne,
13
prevention and, 147
principles of, 63
and seriousness of acne, 16
see also medications
tretinoin (retinoic acid), 59, 63,
69–71, 81–82, 155
trichloroacetic acid (TCA), 181
triclosan, 52, 207
tropical acne, 44

ultraviolet light, 29, 87
acne caused by, 43
looking good and, 156–57
prescription treatments and, 70,
74, 85

Vaseline, 103
vellus follicles, 19
Vietnam War, 44
vitamins, 210
A, 59–60, 67, 74, 92–94, 103,
126–27, 129
B complex, 86, 126, 128, 134
C, 126, 128–29
CAM and, 126–29, 134
E, 126, 128–29, 134
VitaNiacin, 134
Vitex, 131

waxing, 104
Webster, Guy, 105
Wexler, Patricia, 15, 17
white blood cells, 132, 136

white blood cells *(cont.)*
  and causes of acne, 43
  see also neutrophils
whiteheads, 33, 110
  acne formation and, 18, 23–24, 26
  CAM and, 134
  and causes of acne, 37
  children and, 165–66, 168
  extraction of, 152–54
  OTC remedies and, 65
  prescription treatments and, 67,
    101–2
working women:
  acne in, 4–5
  mind-skin connection and, 139,
    145

World Congress of Dermatology,
  100
World War II, 44

Yarborough, John, 91, 185, 193
Yasmin, 116–17
yeast infections, 78, 165

ZAPZYT, 207–8, 210, 212
zinc, 127, 129
  prescription treatments and, 83,
    86
  topical, 136
zinc oxide, 157
Zyderm, 189–90
Zyplast, 189–90